THE SCIENCE STUDY SERIES

The Science Study Series originated as part of the Physical Science Study Committee (of Educational Services Incorporated, now Education Development Center) program for the teaching and study of physics. The Series offers to students and to the general public the writing of distinguished authors on the most stirring and fundamental topics of science, from the smallest known particles to the whole universe. Some of the books tell of the role of science in the world of man, his technology and civilization. Others are biographical in nature, telling the fascinating stories of the great discoverers and their discoveries. All of the authors have been selected both for expertise in the fields they discuss and for ability to communicate their special knowledge and their own views in an interesting way. The primary purpose of these books is to provide a survey within the grasp of the young student or the layman. Many of the books, it is hoped, will encourage the reader to make his own investigations of natural phenomena.

The Speech Chain

PETER B. DENES obtained his Bachelor's and Master's Degrees in Electrical Engineering from the University of Manchester and his Ph.D. in Engineering from the University of London. From 1946–61 he served as lecturer in experimental phonetics and head of the laboratory of the Phonetics Department at University College, London. During that period, he also held an appointment as part-time physicist at the Audiology Unit, Royal National Throat, Nose and Ear Hospital, and was a member of the Medical and Scientific Committee, Royal National Institute for the Deaf.

After coming to the United States in 1961, he joined Bell Telephone Laboratories, becoming Head of the Speech and Communication Research Department in 1967. Dr. Denes' research interests have been primarily concerned with the nature of the human speech process and with improved man-computer communication.

Dr. Denes is a Fellow of the Acoustical Society of America, Ex-Chairman of its Committee on Speech Communication, and Associate Editor of the Journal of the Acoustical Society of America. He is the author or co-author of many articles concerned with speech research, hearing tests, and hearing aids.

ELLIOT N. PINSON was born in New York City. After graduating *summa cum laude* from Princeton in 1956 he attended MIT on a Whiton Fellowship, receiving his Master's Degree in 1957. He continued his studies in electrical engineering at the California Institute of Technology, and his research on adaptive control systems led to a Ph.D. in 1961.

Dr. Pinson joined the Technical Staff of Bell Telephone Laboratories in 1961, where he engaged in research on speech analysis and synthesis and, later, computer graphics. He is currently Head of the Computer Systems Research Department where his chief interests are research on computer architecture, computer networks, and operating systems.

Dr. Pinson was an Instructor in Electrical Engineering at Cal Tech during 1960–61, and was visiting Mackay Lecturer in the Electrical Engineering and Computer Sciences Department at the University of California, Berkeley, during 1969–70. He is a member of Phi Beta Kappa and Sigma Xi and the author or co-author of several papers on speech analysis and computer systems.

The Speech Chain

THE PHYSICS AND BIOLOGY
OF SPOKEN LANGUAGE

PETER B. DENES

ELLIOT N. PINSON

Bell Telephone Laboratories

ANCHOR PRESS/DOUBLEDAY
GARDEN CITY, NEW YORK.

1973

Anchor Science Study Series
edition published in 1973.

Copyright © 1963 by Bell Telephone Laboratories, Incorporated
ISBN: 0-385-04237-X

Library of Congress Catalog Number 63–18609

Printed in the United States of America

PREFACE

A striking characteristic of our century is the rapid expansion of science. It is no longer possible for a person to have an up-to-date familiarity with all fields. New knowledge is being brought to light—and new fields explored—at a rate that makes it difficult for scientists and engineers to keep abreast of developments in their own fields, let alone those outside their immediate concern.

Inevitably, this creates problems for the men and women responsible for setting school curricula. The teaching time available is not sufficient to cover all subjects. The usual approach is to present formal courses on several broad disciplines, like physics, biology and history. Each subject is presented independently and there is little time to show their interrelation.

Of course, many subjects do not fall wholly within any one of the established categories. Communication by speech is such a subject. Its understanding requires a knowledge of anatomy, physiology, physics, psychology and linguistics. It provides an excellent illustration of the interrelation of concepts from a wide range of disciplines, and it shows to advantage what can be gained by using the points of view and methods of investigation of several disciplines.

Spoken communication is not only an interdisciplinary subject; it is also an extremely important human activity. It sets us apart from other animals and is closely related to our power of reasoning. In addition, it is the most commonly used form of communication and has influenced the way human societies have developed.

This book—presenting a significant subject in an interdisciplinary manner—should be suitable for good high school students at the junior or senior grades and, perhaps, for certain college students as well. We hope that any student interested in spoken communication will find the text understandable and rewarding, whether his primary interest is physics, biology or the humanities. We have certainly tried to present the material in a way understandable to all, without requiring previous knowledge of the fields involved.

We do not give a detailed account of our subject. The selection of topics rested to a great extent on the particular interests of the authors and, of course, on what we thought was important.

The authors are grateful to those who helped in the preparation of this book. We owe a special debt to D. H. Van Lenten, whose fine editing improved the readability of the book. His efforts to coordinate the work of the authors also were invaluable.

J. L. Flanagan and E. E. David read the entire

manuscript and made many valuable suggestions. Others who have helped us on one or more chapters include L. D. Harmon, N. Guttman, W. van Bergeijk, M. Sondhi, Stefi Pinson, and Joan Miller, who programmed a computer to generate some of the illustrations.

We have rarely given credit in the body of the text to those scientists whose work we describe. We felt that annotations and footnotes would detract from the readability of our presentation. An annotated reading list is given at the end of the book, where the interested reader can find publications that go more deeply than we have into various aspects of spoken communication.

PETER B. DENES
ELLIOT N. PINSON

PREFACE TO THE REVISED EDITION

The Speech Chain was first published in 1963 as one part of a continuing Bell System program to provide educational aids for secondary-school science programs. The authors were gratified by the enthusiastic response which it received. It has since gone through six printings with a total distribution of about 100,000 copies. These books have been distributed primarily through Operating Telephone Companies, although an appreciable number were purchased by readers directly from the supplier. Happily, the demand for the book, despite the fact that it was publicized very little, has outstripped the distribution system which has up to now prevailed. We are very pleased, therefore, that this new edition of *The Speech Chain* is available through normal publishing and distribution channels.

We gave a good deal of thought to the desirability of an extensive revision of the book to include new material on techniques which have become important in speech and hearing research. These include primarily the great advances that have been made in using computers for a variety of tasks including speech synthesis, automation of acoustic experiments, and modeling various aspects of the speech chain. In rereading the text, it did not seem feasible to improve the book without substantially increasing its size. This would be likely to change the flavor and usefulness of the product in an unknown way. Rather than take that risk, we have decided to reissue *The Speech Chain* essentially unchanged. The annotated reading list at the end of the book has been expanded and updated to some extent, and we have made corrections in the figures and text where errors have been discovered.

Although *The Speech Chain* was conceived originally for a secondary-school audience, we hoped that it would appeal to a broader audience as well. We have been pleased by the fact that a large number of our readers are college students in courses on phonetics, linguistics, and speech therapy. We hope *The Speech Chain* will continue to fill a need for scientific information in these interdisciplinary fields.

P. B. DENES
E. N. PINSON

Murray Hill, N.J., 1972

Contents

CHAPTER 1. The Speech Chain   1

A discussion of the different forms in which a
spoken message exists in its progress from the
mind of the speaker to the mind of the listener; linguistic, physiological, anatomical and
acoustic aspects of speech production and perception.

CHAPTER 2. Linguistic Organization   13

The phoneme, the syllable, the word and the
sentence; grammatical and semantic rules of
linguistic organization; stress and intonation.

CHAPTER 3. The Physics of Sound   19

Vibrations; free and forced vibrations; resonance; frequency response; sound waves in air;
Fourier's theorem; the spectrum; sound pres-

sure; sound intensity; the decibel scale; acoustical resonance.

CHAPTER 4. Speech Production   51

The anatomy of the vocal organs: lungs, trachea, larynx, pharynx, nose and mouth; the movement of vocal organs during speech; the vibration of the vocal cords; the articulatory movements of the tongue, lips, teeth and soft palate; articulatory description of English speech sounds; the articulatory classification of vowels and consonants; the acoustics of speech production: formants, the spectra of speech sounds.

CHAPTER 5. Hearing   85

Anatomy and physiology of hearing: the outer ear, the middle ear, the inner ear, the cochlea, the Organ of Corti; the perception of sound: hearing acuity, loudness and intensity, pitch and frequency, differential thresholds, masking effects, binaural effects.

CHAPTER 6. Nerves, Brain and The
            Speech Chain   121

Neurons; nerve impulses; peripheral and central nervous systems; thought and speech; hearing and the nervous system; theories of hearing.

CHAPTER 7. The Acoustic
Characteristics of Speech 149

The intensities of speech waves; the spectra
of speech waves; the formants of English
vowels; the sound spectrograph; spectrograms
of continuous speech; visible speech and its
use in teaching deaf children.

CHAPTER 8. Speech Recognition 163

The measurement of speech intelligibility;
acoustic cues for speech recognition; vowel recognition; experiments with artificial speech;
the Pattern-Playback; plosive bursts; formant
transitions; fricatives; duration as a cue for
recognition; experiments with natural speech;
non-acoustic cues; speech recognition—the result of acoustic, linguistic and other contextual cues.

CHAPTER 9. A Look Toward
the Future 193

Speaker identification; speech recognition;
speech synthesis; bandwidth compression systems; advances in neurophysiology; the path of
scientific research.

READING LIST 205

INDEX 209

The Speech Chain

Chapter 1

THE SPEECH CHAIN

We usually take for granted our ability to produce and understand speech and give little thought to its nature and function, just as we are not particularly aware of the action of our hearts, brains, or other essential organs. It is not surprising, therefore, that many people overlook the great influence of speech on the development and normal functioning of human society.

Wherever human beings live together, they develop a system of talking to each other; even people in the most primitive societies use speech. Speech, in fact, is one of those few, basic abilities—tool making is another—that set us apart from animals and are closely connected with our ability to think abstractly.

Why is speech so important? One reason is that the development of human civilization is made possible—to a great extent—by man's ability to share experiences, to exchange ideas and to transmit knowledge from one generation to another; in other words, his ability to communicate with other men. We can communicate with each other in many ways. The smoke signals of the Apache Indian, the starter's pistol in a 100-yard dash, the finger signing language used by deaf people, the Morse Code and various systems of writing are just a few examples of the many different systems of communication developed by man. Unquestionably, however, speech is the system that man has found to be far more efficient and convenient than any other.

You may think that writing is a more important means of communication. After all, the development of civilization and the output of printing presses seem to parallel each other, and the written word appears to be a more efficient and more durable means of transmitting intelligence. It must be remembered, however, that no matter how many books and newspapers are printed, the amount of intelligence exchanged by speech is still vastly greater. The widespread use of books and printed matter may very well be an indication of a highly developed civilization, but so is the greater use of telephone systems. Those areas of the world where civilization is most highly developed are also the areas with the greatest density of telephones; and countries bound by social and political ties are usually connected by a well developed telephone system.

We can further bolster our argument that speech has a more fundamental influence than writing on the development of civilization by citing the many human societies that have developed and flourished without evolving a system of reading and writing. We know of no civilization, however, where speech was not available.

Perhaps the best example of the overwhelming importance of speech in human society is a comparison of the social attitudes of the blind to those of the deaf. Generally, blind people tend to get along with their fellow human beings despite their handicap. But the deaf, who can still read and write, often feel cut off from society. A deaf person, deprived of his primary means of communication, tends to withdraw from the world and live within himself.

In short, human society relies heavily on the free and easy interchange of ideas among its members and, for one reason or another, man has found speech to be his most convenient form of communication.

Through its constant use as a tool essential to daily living, speech has developed into a highly efficient system for the exchange of even our most complex ideas. It is a system particularly suitable for widespread use under the constantly changing and varied conditions of life. It is suitable because it remains functionally unaffected by the many different voices, speaking habits, dialects and accents of the millions who use a common language. And it is suitable for widespread use because speech—to a surprising extent—is invulnerable to severe noise, distortion and interference.

Speech is well worth careful study. It is worthwhile because the study of speech provides useful insights into the nature and history of human civilization. It is worthwhile for the communications engineer because a better understanding of the speech mechanisms enables him to exploit its built-in features in developing better and more efficient communication systems. It is worthwhile for all of us because we depend on speech so heavily for communicating with others.

The study of speech is also important in the just-emerging field of man-to-machine communication. We all use automatons, like the dial telephone and automatic elevator, which either get their instructions from us or report back to us on their operations. Frequently, they do both, like the highly complex digital computers used in scientific laboratories. In designing communication systems or "languages" to link man and machine, it may prove especially worthwhile to have a firm understanding of speech, that system of man-to-man communication whose development is based on the experience of many generations.

When most people stop to consider speech, they think only in terms of moving lips and tongue. A few others who have found out about sound waves, perhaps in the course of building hi-fi sets, will also associate certain kinds of sound waves with speech. In reality, speech is a far more complex process, involving many more levels of human activity, than such a simple approach would suggest.

A convenient way of examining what happens during speech is to take the simple situation of two people talking to each other; one of them, the speaker, transmits information to the other, the listener. The first thing the speaker has to do is arrange his thoughts, decide what he wants to say and put what he wants to say into *linguistic form*. The message is put into linguistic form by selecting the right words and phrases to express its meaning, and by placing these words in the correct order required by the grammatical rules of the language. This process is associated with activity in the speaker's brain, and it is in the brain that appropriate instructions, in the form of impulses along the motor nerves, are sent to the muscles of the vocal organs, the tongue, the lips and the vocal cords. The nerve impulses set the vocal muscles into movement which, in turn, produces minute pressure changes in the surrounding air. We call these pressure changes a sound wave.

The movements of the vocal organs generate a speech sound wave that travels through the air between speaker and listener. Pressure changes at the ear activate the listener's hearing mechanism and produce nerve impulses

THE SPEECH CHAIN

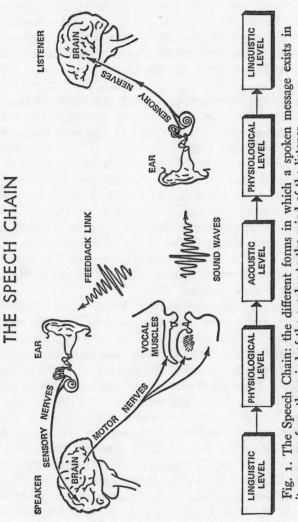

Fig. 1. The Speech Chain: the different forms in which a spoken message exists in its progress from the mind of the speaker to the mind of the listener.

that travel along the acoustic nerve to the listener's brain. In the listener's brain, a considerable amount of nerve activity is already taking place, and this activity is modified by the nerve impulses arriving from the ear. This modification of brain activity, in ways we do not fully understand, brings about recognition of the speaker's message. We see, therefore, that speech communications consists of a chain of events linking the speaker's brain with the listener's brain. We shall call this chain of events *the speech chain*. (See Fig. 1.)

It might be worthwhile to mention at this point that the speech chain has an important side link. In the simple speaker-listener situation just described, there are really two listeners, not one, because the speaker not only speaks, he also listens to his own voice. In listening, he continuously compares the quality of the sounds he produces with the sound qualities he intended to produce and makes the adjustments necessary to match the results with his intentions.

There are many ways to show that a speaker is his own listener. Perhaps the most amusing is to delay the sound "fed back" to the speaker. This can be done quite simply by recording the speaker's voice on a tape recorder and playing it back a fraction of a second later. The speaker listens to the delayed version over earphones. Under such circumstances, the unexpected delay in the fed-back sound makes the speaker stammer and slur. This is the so-called *delayed speech feedback effect*. Another example of the importance of "feedback" is the general deterioration of the speech of people who have suffered prolonged deafness. Deafness, of course, deprives these people of the speech chain's feedback link. To some limited extent, we can tell the kind of deafness from the type of speech deterioration it produces.

Let us go back now to the main speech chain, the links

that connect speaker with listener. We have seen that the transmission of a message begins with the selection of suitable words and sentences. This can be called the *linguistic level* of the speech chain.

The speech event continues on the *physiological level*, with neural and muscular activity, and ends, on the speaker's side, with the generation and transmission of a sound wave, the *physical level* of the speech chain.

At the listener's end of the chain, the process is reversed. Events start on the physical level, when the incoming sound wave activates the hearing mechanism. They continue on the physiological level with neural activity in the hearing and perceptual mechanisms. The speech chain is completed on the linguistic level when the listener recognizes the words and sentences transmitted by the speaker. The speech chain, therefore, involves activity on at least three different levels, the linguistic, physiological and physical, first on the speaker's side and then at the listener's end.

We may also think of the speech chain as a communication system in which ideas to be transmitted are represented by a code that undergoes transformations as speech events proceed from one level to another. We can draw an analogy here between speech and Morse code. In Morse code, certain patterns of dots and dashes stand for different letters of the alphabet; the dots and dashes are a code for the letters. This code can also be transformed from one form to another. For example, a series of dots and dashes on a piece of paper can be converted into an acoustic sequence, like "beep-bip-bip-beep." In the same way, the words of our language are a code for concepts and material objects. The word "dog" is the code for a four-legged animal that wags its tail, just as "dash-dash-dash" is Morse code for the letter "O." We learn the code words of a language—and the rules for combining them into sentences—when we learn to speak.

During speech transmission, the speaker's linguistic code of words and sentences is transformed into physiological and physical codes—in other words, into corresponding sets of muscle movements and air vibrations—before being reconverted into a linguistic code at the listener's end. This is analogous to translating the written "dash-dash-dash" of Morse code into the sounds, "beep-beep-beep."

Although we can regard speech transmission as a chain of events in which a code for certain ideas is transformed from one level or medium to another, it would be a great mistake to think that corresponding events at the different levels are the same. There is some relationship, to be sure, but the events are far from being identical. For example, there is no guarantee that people will produce sound waves with identical characteristics when they pronounce the same word. In fact, they are more likely to produce sound waves of different characteristics when they pronounce the same word. By the same token, they may very well generate similar sound waves when pronouncing different words.

This state of affairs was clearly demonstrated in an experiment carried out a few years ago. A group of people listened to the same sound wave, representing a word, on three occasions when the word was used in three different-sounding sentences. The listeners agreed that the test word was either "bit" or "bet" or "bat," depending on which of the three sentences was used.

The experiment clearly shows that the general circumstances (context) under which we listen to speech profoundly affect the kind of words we associate with particular sound waves. In other words, the relationship between a word and a particular sound wave, or between a word and a particular muscle movement or pattern of nerve impulses, is not unique. There is no label on a speech sound wave that invariably associates it with a particular word. Depending on context, we recognize a particular sound wave as one word or another. A good example of this is reported by people who speak several languages fluently. They sometimes recognize indistinctly heard phrases as being spoken in one of their languages, but realize later that the conversation was in another of their languages.

Knowledge of the right context can even make the difference between understanding and not understanding a particular sound wave sequence. You probably know that at some airports you can pay a dime and listen in on the conversations between pilots and the control tower. The chances are that many of the sentences would be incomprehensible to you because of noise and distortion. Yet this same speech wave would be clearly intelligible to the pilots simply because they have more knowledge of context than you. In this case, the context is provided by their experience in listening under conditions of distortion, and by their greater knowledge of the kind of messages to expect.

The strong influence of circumstance on what you recognize is not confined to speech. When you watch television or movies, you probably consider the scenes you see as quite life-like. But pictures on television are much smaller than life-size and much larger on a movie screen. Context will make the small television picture, the life-sized original and the huge movie scene appear to be the same size. Black-and-white television and movies also appear quite life-like, despite their lack of true color. Once again, context makes the multicolored original and the black and white screen seem similar. In speech, as in these examples, we are quite unaware of our heavy reliance on context.

We can say, therefore, that speakers will not generally produce identical sound waves when they pronounce the same words on different occasions. The listener, in recognizing speech, does not rely solely on information derived from the speech wave he receives. He also relies on his knowledge of an intricate communication system subject to the rules of language and speech, and on cues provided by the subject matter and the identity of the speaker.

In speech communication, then, we do not actually rely on a precise knowledge of specific cues. Instead, we relate a great variety of ambiguous cues against the background of the complex system we call our common language. When you think about it, there is really no other way speech could function efficiently. It does seem unlikely that millions of speakers, with all their different voice qualities, speaking habits and accents, would ever produce anything like identical sound waves when they say the same words. People engaged in speech research know this only too well, much to their regret. Even though our instruments for measuring the characteristics of sound waves are considerably more accurate and flexible than the human ear, we are still unable to build a machine that will recognize speech. We can measure characteristics of speech waves with great accuracy, but we do not know the nature and rules of the contextual system against which the results of our measurements must be related, as they are so successfully related in the brains of listeners.

In the following chapters, we will describe the speech chain—from speaker to listener—as fully as our knowledge and the scope of this book allow. What we have said so far should give you some clues as to why only a part of what follows is concerned with the laws governing events on any one level of the speech chain; in other words, with the physics of speech and the behavior of nerves and muscles. The rest of the book, in common with the dominant trends of modern speech research, deals with the relationship of events on different levels of the speech chain, and how the events are affected by context. It describes the kinds of sound waves produced when we speak the speech sounds and words of English; the relationship between the articulatory movements of our vocal organs and the speech wave produced; how our hearing mechanism transforms sound waves into nerve impulses and sensations; and how we perceive and recognize speech sound waves as words and sentences. The final chapter discusses some of the practical uses to which the results of speech research are applied, and the aims and methods of research now in progress.

Chapter 2

LINGUISTIC ORGANIZATION

In our discussion of the nature of speech, we explained that the message to be transmitted from speaker to listener is first arranged in linguistic form; the speaker chooses the right words and sentences to express what he wants to say. The information then goes through a series of transformations into physiological and acoustic forms, and is finally reconverted into linguistic form at the listener's end. The listener fits his auditory sensations into a sequence of words and sentences; the process is completed when he understands what the speaker said.

Throughout the rest of this book, we will concern ourselves with relating events on the physiological and acoustic levels with events on the linguistic level. When describing speech production, we will give an account of the type of vocal organ movements associated with speech sounds and words. When describing speech recognition, we will discuss the kinds of speech sounds and words perceived when we hear sound waves with particular acoustic features. In this chapter, we will concentrate on what happens on the linguistic level itself; we will concentrate, in other words, on describing the units of language and how they function.

The units of language are symbols. Many of these symbols stand for objects around us and for familiar concepts and ideas. Words, for example, are symbols: the word "table" is the symbol for an object we use in our homes, the word "happy" represents a certain state of mind, and so on. Language is a system consisting of these symbols and the rules for combining them into sequences that express our thoughts, our intentions and our experiences. Learning to speak and understand a language involves learning these symbols, together with the rules for assembling them in the right order. We spend much of the first few years of our lives learning the rules of our native language. Through practice, they become habitual, and we can apply them without being conscious of their influence.

The most familiar language units are words. Words, however, can be thought of as sequences of smaller linguistic units, the *speech sounds* or *phonemes*. The easiest way to understand the nature of phonemes is to consider a group of words like "heed," "hid," "head" and "had." We instinctively regard such words as being made up of an initial, a middle and a final element. In our four examples, the initial and final elements are identical, but the middle elements are different; it is the difference in this middle element that distinguishes the four words. Similarly, we can compare all the words of a language and find those sounds that differentiate one word from another. Such distinguishing sounds are called phonemes and they are the basic linguistic units from which words and sentences are put together. Phonemes on their own do not symbolize any concept or object; only in relation to other phonemes do they distinguish one word from another. The phoneme "p," for example, has no independent meaning, but in combination with other phonemes, it can distinguish "heat" from "heap," "peel" from "keel," and so forth.

We can divide phonemes into two groups, vowels or consonants, depending on their position in larger linguistic units (to be explained below). There are 16 vowels and 22 consonants in English, as listed in Table I.

TABLE I—THE PHONEMES OF GENERAL AMERICAN ENGLISH

General American is the dialect of English spoken in midwestern and western areas of the United States and influences an increasing number of Americans. Certain phonemes of other regional dialects (e.g. Southern) can be different.

Vowels	Consonants	
ee as in *heat*	*t* as in *tee*	*s* as in *see*
I as in *hit*	*p* as in *pea*	*sh* as in *shell*
e as in *head*	*k* as in *key*	*h* as in *he*
ae as in *had*	*b* as in *bee*	*v* as in *view*
ah as in *father*	*d* as in *dawn*	*th* as in *then*
aw as in *call*	*g* as in *go*	*z* as in *zoo*
U as in *put*	*m* as in *me*	*zh* as in *garage*
oo as in *cool*	*n* as in *no*	*l* as in *law*
ʌ as in *ton*	*ng* as in *sing*	*r* as in *red*
uh as in *the*	*f* as in *fee*	*y* as in *you*
er as in *bird*	*θ* as in *thin*	*w* as in *we*
oi as in *toil*		
au as in *shout*		
ei as in *take*		
ou as in *tone*		
ai as in *might*		

Phonemes can be combined into larger units called *syllables*. Although linguists do not always agree on the definition of a syllable, most native speakers of English have an instinctive feeling for its nature. A syllable usually has a vowel for a central phoneme, surrounded by one or more consonants. In most languages, there are restrictions on the way phonemes may be combined into larger units.

In English, for example, we never find syllables that start with an "ng" phoneme: syllables like "ngees" or "ngoot" are impossible. Of course, such rules reduce the variety of syllables used in a language; the total number of English syllables is between only one and two thousand.

An even larger linguistic unit is the *word*, which normally consists of a sequence of several phonemes and one or more syllables. The most frequently used English words are sequences of between two and five phonemes. There are some words, like "awe" and "a," which have only one phoneme, and others that are made up of 10 or more phonemes.

The most frequently used words are, on the whole, short words with just a few phonemes. This suggests that economy of speaking effort may have an influence on the way language develops. Table II shows the 10 most frequently used English words.

TABLE II—THE TEN MOST FREQUENTLY USED WORDS IN ENGLISH

I	you
the	of
a	and
it	in
to	he

Only a very small fraction of possible phoneme combinations are used as words in English. Even so, there are several hundred thousand English words, and new ones are being added every day. Although the total number of words is very large, only a few thousand are frequently used. Various language surveys indicate that—95 per cent of the time—we choose words from a library of only 5000 to 10,000 words. The vast number of other words are rarely used.

Words are combined into still longer linguistic units called *sentences*. The rules that outline the way sequences of words can be combined to form acceptable sentences are called the *grammar* of a language. Grammar tells us that the string of words, "the plants are green," is acceptable, but the sequence, "plants green are the," is not.

Grammar alone, however, does not determine word order. Sentences must make sense as well as satisfy the rules of grammar. For example, a sentence like "the horse jumped over the fence" is both grammatically acceptable and sensible. But the sequence, "the strength jumped over the fence," although grammatically correct, is meaningless and does not occur in normal use. The study of word meanings is called *semantics,* and we can see from our two examples that word order is influenced both by grammatical and semantic considerations.

Stress and *intonation* are also part of linguistic organization. They are used to express such things as the speaker's emotional attitude, to make distinctions between questions, statements and doubt, etc., and to indicate the relative importance attached to different words in a sentence. We can, for example, alter the sense of identical sentences simply by using stress and intonation. We can say, "I will be the judge of that" or "I will be the judge of *that,*" and, although the same words appear in the two sequences, the meanings of the two sentences are dissimilar. Stress and intonation are used extensively during speech, but there is really no adequate method of representing them in written material. We can use different types of punctuation, but this is only a partial solution of the problem. In fact, the trouble we occasionally have—when writing—to indicate distinctions quite easy to make in speech by stress and intonation, is a good example of their importance.

We have now seen that the fundamental units of our linguistic system are the phonemes, the words, and so forth. In addition, we have the grammatical and semantic rules for combining these units into longer sequences. Stress and intonation are also important aspects of language. Together, they form the linguistic basis of speech, our most commonly used communication system.

In a later chapter, we will discuss the considerable influence of linguistics on speech recognition; we will see how linguistic rules make speech the highly flexible and versatile communication system it is.

Chapter 3

THE PHYSICS OF SOUND

Before we can discuss the nature of speech sound waves
—how they are produced and perceived—we must understand a certain amount about sound waves in general.
Sound waves in air are the principal subject of this
chapter. The subject forms part of the field of *acoustics*.
Since our book is concerned with the broad topic of
spoken communication, we will present only a brief introduction to the physics of sound, with emphasis on
those aspects that are necessary for understanding the
material in following chapters.

Sound waves in air are just one example of a large class
of physical phenomena that involve *wave motion*. Surface
waves in water and electromagnetic radiations, like radio
waves and light, are other examples. All wave motion is
produced by—and consists of—the vibration of certain
quantities. In the case of sound waves, air particles are
set into vibration; in the case of surface waves in water,
water particles; and in the case of electromagnetic waves,
the electrical and magnetic fields associated with the wave

oscillate rapidly. Since vibrations play such an important part in wave motion, we will begin by explaining a few elementary facts about them.

VIBRATION

Perhaps the best way to approach the subject of vibration is in terms of a simple example. There are many to choose from, such as the vibrating prongs of a tuning fork, an oscillating piano string, a pendulum, or a spring and mass.

Let us examine the spring and mass arrangement shown in Fig. 2. One end of the spring is rigidly fixed and cannot move; the other end is attached to the mass, say a metal block. The mass rests on a surface it can easily slide along. When it is in its normal resting position, the pointer attached to the mass is at position B on the ruler.

If the mass is moved toward point A, the spring will be compressed and will exert a force on the mass that tends to move it back toward its rest position. If the mass is moved in the other direction, toward point C, the spring will be stretched; again, a force will act on the

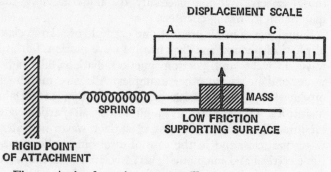

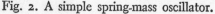

Fig. 2. A simple spring-mass oscillator.

mass, tending to make it move toward its rest position, B. We see, then, that the spring always exerts a "restoring force" that tends to move the mass toward its rest position.

Suppose we displace the mass, say to point A, and release it. The spring force will make the mass move toward B. It will gain speed until it reaches point B and, because of its *inertia*, will pass through its rest position. Inertia, a property common to all matter, causes a body in motion to remain in motion (or a body at rest to remain at rest) in the absence of external forces. Once the mass is on the right-hand side of its rest position, the spring's restoring force opposes its motion and, eventually, brings it to a stop. The mass is again set in motion by the spring force acting in the direction of the rest position; it will pass through its rest position and continue to move back and forth. This to and fro motion of a body about its rest position is called *oscillation* or *vibration*.

Vibrations are likely to occur whenever the two properties of *mass* and *elasticity* ("springiness") are present together. In air, the individual molecules are the masses of the system. The forces that act between these molecules behave very much like spring forces. For example, if we try to pack an excess number of molecules into a limited volume, a force arises that tends to resist the compression. This is the force that keeps a balloon or tire inflated and opposes our efforts to inflate a bicycle tire with a hand pump. These forces resemble spring behavior.

PROPERTIES OF VIBRATING SYSTEMS

All types of vibration have certain basic properties in common. We will define these properties, using as our example the spring-mass system of Fig. 2. These definitions apply to all vibratory motions and will be extensively used later in connection with sound waves. First, we will describe what we mean by the *amplitude, frequency* and *period* of a vibration.

If the mass is displaced from its rest position and allowed to vibrate, it moves back and forth between two positions that mark the extreme limits of its motion. The distance of the mass from point B at any instant is called its *displacement.* The maximum displacement is called the *amplitude* of the vibration. If there are no energy losses during the motion—due to friction, for example— the maximum displacement of the mass will be the same on both sides of its rest position. Furthermore, the size of the displacement will be the same each successive time the mass moves out to the extremes of its motion.

The movement of the mass from A to C and back to A is called one *cycle* of oscillation. The number of complete cycles that take place in one second is called the *frequency* of the oscillation. If 15 complete cycles occur in one second, we say that the vibration has a frequency of 15 cycles per second (abbreviated, cps). The sound waves we will be interested in have frequencies ranging from tens to thousands of cycles per second.

The time taken to complete one cycle of vibration is called the *period* of the vibration. There is a simple relationship between the frequency of an oscillation and its period. The frequency is simply 1 *divided by the period;* for example, if the period is $\frac{1}{20}$ of a second, the frequency is 20 cps.

So far, we have more or less assumed that, once set into motion, the spring-mass combination would continue to vibrate indefinitely with the same amplitude. This type of motion is displayed graphically in Fig. 3(a). Here, we show the motion of a spring-mass system that vibrates with a period of two seconds. Initially, the mass is displaced a distance of one inch and released. After its initial displacement, the mass continues to move back and forth between the extremes of its displacement, one inch on either side of its rest position. Consequently, the amplitude of vibration is one inch.

In actual fact, the amplitude of vibration will steadily decrease because of energy losses in the system (due to friction, etc.). Vibrations whose amplitudes decay slowly are said to be lightly "damped," while those whose amplitudes decay rapidly are heavily "damped." Fig. 3(b) and (c) show damped oscillations; the damping is greater in (c).

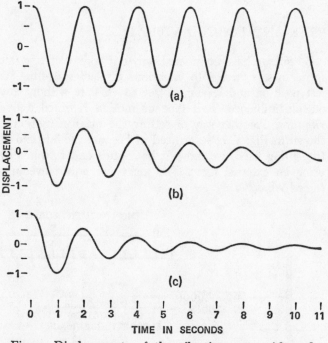

Fig. 3. Displacements of the vibrating mass with and without damping: (a) no loss; (b) lightly damped; (c) more heavily damped.

We will find that the pressure variations that correspond to many interesting acoustic signals—speech waves, for example—are much more complex than the simple shape shown in Fig. 3(a). Nonetheless, we frequently find it convenient to discuss vibrations of this particular form; they are called *sinusoidal* vibrations. The displacement of the mass in our spring-mass system is one example of sinusoidal motion; the movement of a simple pendulum is another. This sort of variation of a quantity with time has important mathematical properties that entitle it to special consideration, as we will see later in this chapter.

FREE AND FORCED VIBRATIONS

So far, we have considered only one way of setting our spring-mass system into vibration: displacing it from its rest position and leaving it free to oscillate without any outside influence. This type of motion is called a *free vibration*. Another way of setting the mass in motion is shown in Fig. 4. Here, instead of keeping the left end of the spring fixed, we move it backwards and forwards by using an external force. The mass will now move in a *forced vibration*.

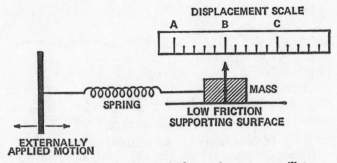

Fig. 4. Forced vibration of the spring-mass oscillator.

In free vibration, for a given mass and spring, the mass will always vibrate sinusoidally (with some damping), and the frequency of the oscillation will always be the same. This characteristic frequency is called its *natural* or *resonant* frequency.

The movement of the mass during a forced vibration depends upon the particular way we move the left-hand end of the spring. In what follows, we will assume that the "driving" motion is a sinusoidal displacement. In this case, the motion of the mass is also sinusoidal. Furthermore, the frequency of vibration of the mass is the same as the frequency of the driving motion.

RESONANCE AND FREQUENCY RESPONSE

If the mass is set into free vibration, in the way previously discussed, the amplitude of the oscillation is determined by the size of the initial displacement. It can be no larger than the initial displacement, and it will decay slowly because of losses in the system. In forced vibration, for a given spring-mass combination, the amplitude of the vibration depends on both the *amplitude* and the *frequency* of the motion impressed on the free end of the spring. For a given amplitude of forcing motion, the vibration of the mass is largest when the driving frequency equals the natural frequency of the system. This phenomenon, whereby a body undergoing forced vibration oscillates with greatest amplitude for applied frequencies near its own natural frequency, is called *resonance*. The frequency at which the maximum response occurs is called the *resonant* frequency, and it is the same as the system's natural frequency.

We can show graphically the amplitude with which the mass oscillates in response to a driving motion of any frequency. Such a graph is called a *frequency response* curve. Two frequency response curves are shown in Fig. 5. The horizontal axis shows the frequency of the driving motion. The vertical axis shows the amplitude of the response (the motion of the mass) for a constant amplitude of applied motion. At 1 cps—the natural frequency of the vibrating body in our example—the response is much larger than the applied motion. This is due to the phenomenon of resonance. The curves in the figure show the behavior of two oscillators having the same natural frequency, but different damping (different amounts of energy loss). The smaller the energy losses, the greater the increase in movement produced by resonance.

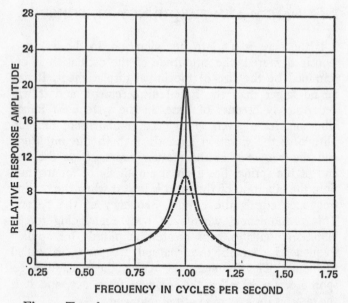

Fig. 5. Two frequency response curves with a resonant frequency of 1 cps. Dashed line shows oscillation with greater damping.

SOUND WAVES IN AIR

All objects on earth are surrounded by air. Air consists of many small particles, more than 400 billion billion in every cubic inch. These particles move about rapidly in random directions. We can explain the generation and propagation of most sound waves without considering such random motions. It is sufficient to assume that each particle has some average "stable" position from which it is displaced by the passage of a sound wave.

If one particle is disturbed—moved nearer some of the others—a force develops that tends to push it back to its original position. Thus, when air is compressed, pushing the particles closer together, a force develops that tends to push them apart. By the same token, when air particles are separated by more than the usual distance, a force develops that tends to push them back into the emptier, rarefied space.

The air particles, in fact, behave just as though they were small masses of matter connected by springs. A line of such particles is shown in the top row of Fig. 6. If we push particle A toward the right, the "spring" between particles A and B is compressed. The spring's increased force will move particle B to the right, in turn increasing the force on the spring between B and C, and so forth. Whenever particles near a certain point are closer together than normal, we say that a state of *compression* exists at that point. The positions of the particles at successive instants of time are shown in the successive rows of Fig. 6. We see that the compression, which started at the left, moves along the line of particles toward the right. Similarly, if we push particle A to the left, we stretch the spring between A and B; the spring tension will move

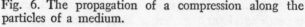

Fig. 6. The propagation of a compression along the particles of a medium.

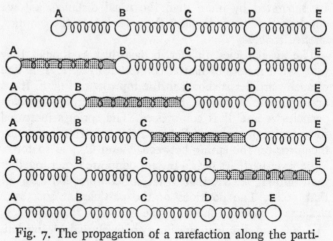

Fig. 7. The propagation of a rarefaction along the particles of a medium.

particle B to the left, stretching the spring between B and C, and so forth. Whenever particles are forced further apart than normal, a state of *rarefaction* is said to exist in their vicinity. Fig. 7 shows that once particle A has been moved to the left, the resulting rarefaction moves toward the right, from particle to particle.

Suppose we have an oscillating tuning fork near particle A, as shown in Fig. 8. Consider what happens when the prong nearest particle A alternately moves it right and left. Each time the prong moves to the right, a compression wave is sent along the particle line; whenever the prong moves to the left, a rarefaction follows the compression wave. The prong moves once to the right and once to the left during each cycle of vibration; consequently, we get a compression followed by a rarefaction along the particle line for every cycle of vibration.

We see that all the particles go through the same back and forth motion as the tuning fork, but that the movement of each particle lags slightly behind the movement of the preceding particle. We also see that only the disturbance itself (the vibration) moves along the line of particles, and that the air particles move back and forth only about their fixed resting positions. A *sound wave* is the movement (propagation) of a disturbance through a material medium such as air, without permanent displacement of the particles themselves.

A simple demonstration can be set up to show that a sound vibration cannot be transmitted in the absence of a material medium. An electric buzzer is placed under a glass jar, as shown in Fig. 9. We can *see* and *hear* the buzzer vibrating. If we now pump the air out of the glass jar, we can *see* that the buzzer continues to vibrate, but the sound we *hear* becomes weaker and weaker as more and more air is removed until, finally, it is inaudible. The

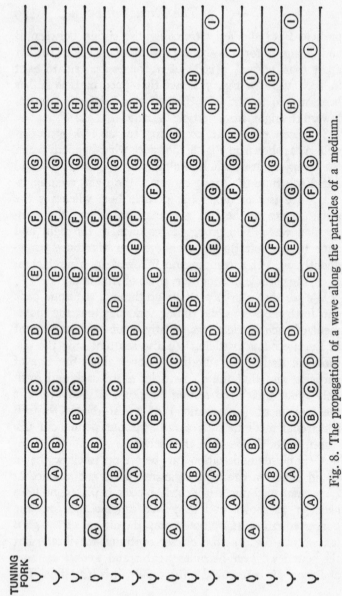

Fig. 8. The propagation of a wave along the particles of a medium.

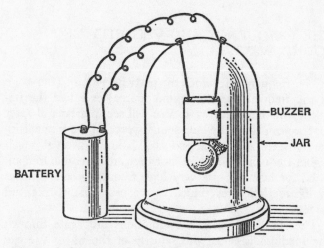

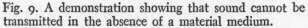

Fig. 9. A demonstration showing that sound cannot be transmitted in the absence of a material medium.

sound will be heard again when air is readmitted to the jar.

Surface waves on water exhibit some of the characteristic features of sound waves. Water waves are vibrations of water particles, much as sound waves are vibrations of air particles. The chief difference between the two is that, in sound waves, the air particles vibrate in the direction of wave movement, while in surface waves, the water particles principally move up and down, at right angles to the direction of wave movement. Instead of the compressions and rarefactions peculiar to sound waves, water waves appear as crests and troughs on the surface of the water.

THE FREQUENCY AND VELOCITY OF A SOUND WAVE

The frequency at which air particles vibrate (the same as the frequency of the sound source) is called the frequency of the sound wave. We will see in a later chapter that we can normally hear sound waves whose frequencies lie between 20 and 20,000 cps. Sound waves at much higher frequencies do exist, but they are inaudible to man. Bats, for instance, use very high frequency sound waves to locate their prey, much as we use radar to pick up targets.

The speed at which the vibrations propagate through the medium is called the *velocity* of the wave. We can determine this velocity in water surface waves by observing the movement of a wave crest. Water waves move slowly, only a few miles an hour. Sound waves in air travel much faster, about 1130 feet per second at sea level; this corresponds to some 770 miles an hour.

How far does the wave travel during one cycle of vibration? We can turn to our tuning fork again. As the fork vibrates, it sends compression after compression along the air particles. The first compression is generated and travels away from the tuning fork; one cycle of vibration later, the fork generates a second compression. By the time the second compression is generated, the first compression has moved further away; the distance between the two compressions is the distance the wave has traveled during one cycle of vibration. The distance between two successive compressions (or between two water wave crests) is called one *wavelength*. A wavelength is also the distance the wave travels in one cycle of vibration of the air particles. If there are f cycles in one second, the wave will travel a distance of f wavelengths in one second. Since the distance traveled in one second is the velocity, it follows that the velocity is equal to the product of the frequency and the wavelength. The wavelength of a sound wave whose frequency is 20 cycles is about 56 feet. If the frequency is increased to 1000 cps, the wavelength becomes shorter—about fourteen inches; at 20,000 cps, the wavelength is slightly less than three-quarters of an inch.

We have already said that every air particle in a sound wave vibrates the same way, except for the time lag between the movements of successive particles. The way a particle vibrates, then, is an important characteristic feature of a sound wave. We can plot the displacement of a particle from its rest position, instant by instant. In sound wave measurement, however, it is usually convenient to measure and plot the sound pressure variations associated with the wave, and not the particle displacement itself. The form of such a curve is called the *waveshape*.

THE SPECTRUM

So far, we have considered only sound waves generated by tuning forks. Tuning forks vibrate sinusoidally and, consequently, the waveshape of the corresponding sound wave is also sinusoidal. Sound waves generated by our vocal organs, however, are almost never sinusoidal. In later chapters, we will see several examples of speech waveshapes; in this chapter, we give only two examples. Fig. 10 shows the typical waveshape of the sound "ah," and Fig. 11 shows the waveshape of the sound "sh." Although the waveshape in Fig. 10 is complicated, it clearly consists of repetitions of the same basic shape. In Fig. 11, on the other hand, there are no such repetitions. The repetitive wave of Fig. 10 is called a *periodic wave*; Fig. 11 shows an *aperiodic* wave. Strictly speaking, only waves with an infinite number of repetitions are periodic. But, in prac-

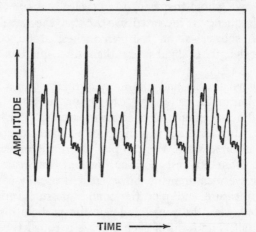

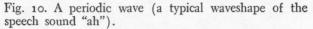

Fig. 10. A periodic wave (a typical waveshape of the speech sound "ah").

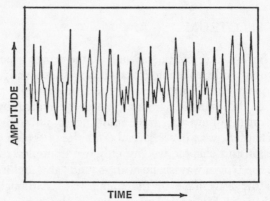

Fig. 11. An aperiodic wave (a typical waveshape of the speech sound "sh").

tice, many speech sound waves have enough repetitions to be regarded as periodic.

The waveshapes of Figs. 10 and 11 are extremely complicated and seem difficult to describe. Fortunately, Joseph Fourier, a French mathematician of the 19th century, showed that any non-sinusoidal wave, no matter how complicated, can be represented as the sum of a number of sinusoidal waves of different frequencies, amplitudes and phases. (The phases of the sinusoidal waves refer to their relative timing—whether they reach the peaks of their vibrations at the same time, for example.) Each of these simple sinusoidal waves is called a *component*.

Fourier's results have been of great importance in analyzing many physical phenomena, not only sound; they were, in fact, originally derived in connection with problems about heat flow in material bodies.

The *spectrum* of the speech wave specifies the amplitudes, frequencies and phases of the wave's sinusoidal components.

The illustrations in Fig. 12 show that the sum of many sinusoidal waves is the equivalent of a wave with a non-sinusoidal shape. The frequencies of the sinusoidal waves in Fig. 12(a) and (b) are, respectively, five and three times the frequency of the wave in (c). When these three waves are added together—just by adding the displacements of all three, instant after instant—we get the clearly non-sinusoidal wave of (d). Notice that the basic pattern of the non-sinusoidal wave repeats with the same periodicity as the lowest frequency component, (c), of all components added.

Fig. 13(a) to (c) shows the same sinusoidal components as Fig. 12(a) to (c), but the phase of the component in Fig. 13(c) is different from the phase of the component in Fig. 12(c). The sum of the three com-

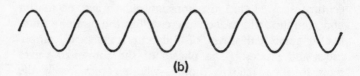

(a)

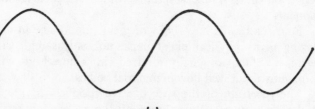

(b)

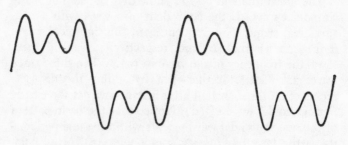

(c)

(d)

Fig. 12. Building up a complex wave: (a), (b) and (c) are sinusoidal components of different frequencies. Portion (a) has five times and portion (b) three times the frequency of portion (c). Portion (d) is the non-sinusoidal sum of (a), (b) and (c).

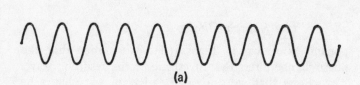

(a)

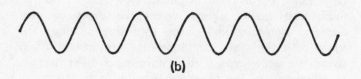

(b)

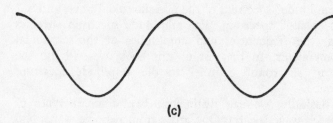

(c)

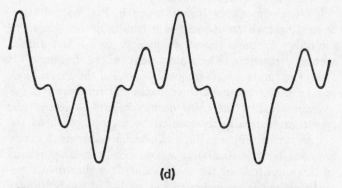

(d)

Fig. 13. The same component waves as shown in Fig. 12 but with the phase of Fig. 12(c) changed; the resulting complex waveform has changed as shown in the (d) portion of this figure.

ponents is shown in Fig. 13(d). We notice that the phase-change alters the waveshape of the resulting wave. This shows that we can get a variety of waveshapes by adding sinusoidal components of the same amplitudes and frequencies, but of different phases. However, our hearing mechanism cannot always detect the effect of such changes. Non-sinusoidal waves, consisting of sinusoidal waves with the same amplitudes and frequencies, often sound the same, even if their waveshapes differ because of differences in the phase relationship of their components. For this reason, we usually consider only the "amplitude" spectrum of the non-sinusoidal wave, and not its "phase" spectrum. The amplitude spectrum specifies just the frequencies and amplitudes of the sinusoidal components. In the rest of this book, we will use the term "spectrum" to refer to the amplitude spectrum alone.

Basically, we can distinguish two different types of speech wave spectra. One arises from periodic waves and the other from aperiodic waves.

For periodic waves (like the one in Fig. 10), the frequency of each component is a whole-number (integer) multiple of some lowest frequency, called the *fundamental frequency*. The component whose frequency is twice the fundamental frequency is called the *second harmonic*; the component three times the fundamental frequency is called the *third harmonic,* and so forth. The spectrum is usually represented by a graph, such as the one shown in Fig. 14. Each sinusoidal component is represented by a vertical line whose height is proportional to the amplitude of the component. It is drawn in a position along the frequency scale—marked at the bottom of the graph—corresponding to the frequency of the component it represents. The higher the frequency of a component, the further to the right we draw the corre-

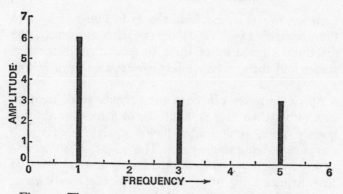

Fig. 14. The spectrum of the complex waves shown in Figs. 12 and 13.

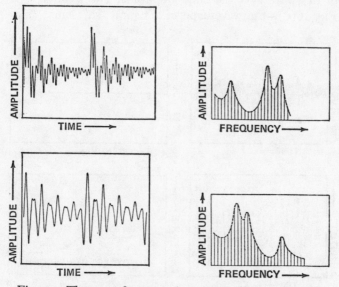

Fig. 15. The waveshapes and corresponding spectra of the vowels "uh" (top) and "ah" (bottom).

sponding line. The spectrum shown in Fig. 14 relates to the wave of Figs. 12(d) or 13(d); consequently, the spectrum is made up of three components. Other waveshapes and their corresponding spectra are shown in Fig. 15.

Aperiodic waves can have components at all frequencies, rather than only at multiples of a fundamental frequency. Thus, we no longer draw a separate line for each component, but a single curve. The height of this curve—at any frequency—represents the energy in the wave near that frequency. Fig. 16(a) shows a typical aperiodic wave; Fig. 16(b) is the corresponding spectrum. It is a horizontal line, indicating that all the spectral components of this wave have the same amplitude. The waveshape of Fig. 16(c)—the waveshape of a typical "sh" sound (also

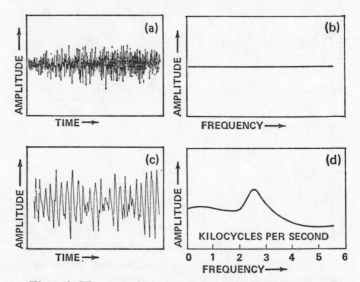

Fig. 16. The waveshapes and corresponding spectra of two different aperiodic waves.

shown in Fig. 14)—is another example of an aperiodic wave. Its corresponding spectrum, Fig. 16(d), has a peak around 2500 cps; this indicates that, of its many components, those in this region are larger in amplitude than the other components.

We have seen that sound waves of any waveshape can be regarded as the sum of a number of waves with simple, sinusoidal shapes. This helps us deal with speech sound waves, which have a great variety of highly non-sinusoidal (complex) waveshapes. In fact, the method is so convenient that we seldom consider the waveshape of the speech wave; that is, we seldom consider the way the sound pressure or deflection of air particles varies with time. Instead, we think in terms of the corresponding spectrum.

We have a convenient and easy-to-use instrument that can measure and display the spectrum of sound waves applied to it. This is the so-called *sound spectrograph*, to be described in Chapter 7.

SOUND PRESSURE AND INTENSITY

Sound Pressure   So far in our description of vibration and wave motion, we have been concerned with the movement of air particles; in other words, with their displacements from their rest positions. The air particles are moved by an external force—like the force exerted by the prongs of a vibrating tuning fork—and each particle exerts force on adjacent particles. The unit of force used most of the time in acoustics is the *dyne*. If, for example, you put a one gram mass—about $\frac{1}{30}$ of an ounce—on the palm of your hand, the gravitational force that tends to push the mass down is equal to about 1000 dynes. *Pressure* is the amount of force acting over a unit area of surface, and the unit of pressure used here is the *dyne per square centimeter*. If, for example, the area of contact between your hand and the one gram mass is two square centimeters, we say that the mass exerts a pressure of about 500 dynes per square centimeter. Normal atmospheric pressure is equal to about one million dynes per square centimeter. In practice, we frequently use units larger than the dyne. For example, we measure tire pressure in pounds per square inch; a tire pressure of 10 pounds per square inch corresponds to a pressure of about 700,000 dynes per square centimeter. The pressures that move air particles—to produce sound waves—are very small. The smallest pressure variation sufficient to produce an audible sound wave is equal to about 0.0002 dynes per square centimeter. At the other end of the scale, sound pressures of 2000 dynes per square centimeter produce sound waves that are not only extremely loud, but strong enough to cause serious damage to the ear.

Sound Intensity   When we push against a heavy stone and move it, we do work or—looking at it another way—we expend energy. When the prongs of a vibrating tuning fork push against an air particle and move it, work is done and energy is expended. Work done is equal to the force exerted on an object, multiplied by the distance the object is moved. A frequently used unit of work and energy is the *erg*. One erg is the amount of work done when a one dyne force displaces an object by one centimeter. Frequently, we are interested in the amount of work done in a given time or, put another way, the rate of doing work. *Power* is the amount of work done in a given time; its unit is the *erg per second*. Since this is much too small for practical use, we normally reckon power in watts or in horsepower. One watt equals 10 million ergs per second, and one horsepower is equal to 746 watts.

In moving surrounding air particles, a vibrating tuning fork transfers a certain amount of energy to them. The air particles, in turn, transfer this energy to more and more air particles as the sound wave spreads out in all directions. The number of air particles affected by the vibrating tuning fork increases with distance from the source; consequently, the amount of energy available to move a particular air particle decreases with distance from the tuning fork. This is why a tuning fork sounds fainter as we move away from it. In measuring the energy levels of sound waves, we are often not interested in the total energy generated by the vibrating source, but only in the energy available over a small area at the point of measurement. The power transmitted along the wave—through an area of one square centimeter at right angles to the direction of propagation—is called the intensity of the sound wave. It is measured in watts per square centimeter. A sound intensity of 10^{-16} watts per square centimeter (one ten thousandth of a millionth of a millionth of one watt per square centimeter) is sufficient to produce a just audible sound; a sound energy of one-hundredth of a watt per square centimeter can damage the ear.

THE DECIBEL SCALE

Most quantities are measured in terms of fixed units. For example, when we say the distance between two points is 20 meters, we mean that the distance between the points is 20 times greater than a one meter length (the reference length of a particular metal rod kept under controlled conditions in Paris). Similarly, when we measure sound intensity in terms of watts per square centimeter, we assume a reference unit of one watt per square centimeter.

Most times, however, it is more convenient to measure sound intensities along the *decibel scale*. Decibels (abbreviated, dB) are not fixed units like watts, grams and meters. When we say that the intensity of a sound wave is one decibel, we only mean that it is a certain number of times greater than some other intensity (about 1.25 times greater). The correct statement is that the sound intensity is one decibel relative to some intensity or another; for example, relative to one watt per square centimeter. The decibel, then, refers to a certain intensity *ratio*. Specifically, the decibel equivalent of a particular *intensity* ratio is 10 times the logarithm to the base 10 of that ratio. It follows from this definition that 10 decibels corresponds to a 10-to-1 intensity ratio. However, 20 deci-

TABLE III—INTENSITY RATIOS AND THEIR DECIBEL EQUIVALENTS

Intensity Ratio		Decibel Equivalent	
1:1		0	
10:1	(the same as 10^1:1)	10	
100:1	(the same as 10^2:1)	20	
1,000:1	(the same as 10^3:1)	30	
10,000:1	(the same as 10^4:1)	40	
100,000:1	(the same as 10^5:1)	50	
1,000,000:1	(the same as 10^6:1)	60	
10,000,000,000:1	(the same as 10^{10}:1)	100	
100,000,000,000,000:1	(the same as 10^{14}:1)	140	
2:1		3	
4:1	(the same as 2 times 2 to 1)	6	(the same as 3 + 3)
8:1	(the same as 4 times 2 to 1)	9	(the same as 6 + 3)
400:1	(the same as 4 times 100 to 1)	26	(the same as 6 + 20)
0.1:1	(the same as 10^{-1}:1)	−10	(minus 10 dB)
0.01:1	(the same as 10^{-2}:1)	−20	
0.4:1	(the same as 0.1 times 4 to 1)	−4	(the same as −10 + 6)

bels *does not* correspond to a 20-fold intensity change. Rather, 20 decibels (10 *plus* 10 decibels) corresponds to a 100-fold (10 *times* 10) intensity change. Table III gives the decibel equivalents of a number of different intensity ratios. The figures in this table immediately show one of the reasons that the decibel scale is so practical. The strongest sounds we can hear without feeling pain are as much as 10 million million times greater in intensity than a just audible sound. This huge intensity ratio corresponds to 130 decibels—a much more convenient figure—on the decibel scale.

Although we can express a sound intensity in decibels relative to any intensity we like, in practice an intensity

TABLE IV—SOUND PRESSURE RATIOS AND
THEIR DECIBEL EQUIVALENTS

Sound Pressure Ratio		Decibel Equivalent	
1:1		0	
10:1	(the same as 10^1:1)	20	
100:1	(the same as 10^2:1)	40	
1,000:1	(the same as 10^3:1)	60	
10,000:1	(the same as 10^4:1)	80	
100,000:1	(the same as 10^5:1)	100	
1,000,000:1	(the same as 10^6:1)	120	
10,000,000:1	(the same as 10^7:1)	140	
2:1		6	
4:1	(the same as 2 times 2 to 1)	12	(the same as 6+6)
8:1	(the same as 4 times 2 to 1)	18	(the same as 12+6)
20:1	(the same as 2 times 10 to 1)	26	(the same as 6+20)
400:1	(the same as 4 times 100 to 1)	52	(the same as 12+40)
0.1:1	(the same as 10^{-1}:1)	−20	(minus 20 dB)
0.01:1	(the same as 10^{-2}:1)	−40	
0.02:1	(the same as 2 times 0.01 to 1)	−34	(the same as +6−40)

of 10^{-16} watts per square centimeter (near the level of a just audible sound) is used most frequently as a reference level. When we find—as we will later—that the average intensity of speech (one meter from the lips) is about 60 decibels relative to 10^{-16} watts per square centimeter, we really mean that this average speech intensity is one million times greater than 10^{-16} watts per square centimeter (see Table III).

It is easier to measure the pressure of a sound wave than its intensity. Consequently, we usually measure the sound pressure and infer the intensity from the pressure value. Sound intensity is proportional to the *square* of the pressure variations of the sound wave. Therefore, a 100-fold increase in intensity produces a 10-fold increase in sound pressure. A 10,000-fold intensity increase corresponds to a 100-fold increase in pressure, and so on. We want the same dB value to apply both to a given intensity ratio and to the corresponding pressure ratio. Consequently, 20 dB must be equivalent to a 10-to-1 pressure ratio (or 100-to-1 intensity ratio). For this reason, the dB equivalent of a particular pressure ratio is 20 times the logarithm to the base 10 of that ratio. The square-law relationship between pressure and intensity explains why the same change in decibels refers to different values of pressure and intensity ratios. Table IV gives the decibel equivalents of a selection of sound pressure ratios.

ACOUSTICAL RESONANCE

We have now discussed the nature of vibration, resonance and sound waves. We will conclude this chapter by explaining acoustical resonance which, as we will see in Chapter 4, plays an extremely important part in speech production.

Enclosed volumes of air can resonate just like the spring-mass combination we described earlier. When a sound wave reaches a volume of air enclosed in a container, an increase in the sound pressure compresses the air in the container. The "springiness" of the air inside the container tends to push the compressed air out again. If the rarefaction of the sound wave reaches the container at the same time the compressed air is being pushed out, the pressure of the sound wave and the pressure of the compressed air will add together and the air particles will move with increased amplitude. If the rate of arrival of the sound wave's compressions and rarefactions (the rate being equal to the sound wave's frequency of vibration) corresponds to a natural frequency of the enclosed air, we get increased movement or *resonance*. When we fill a bottle with water, we can actually *hear* it filling up. Resonance explains this: the splashing water generates sounds of many different frequencies, but the resonance of the air column above the water level emphasizes only those frequencies in the sound that are near its own natural frequency. As the bottle fills up, the size of the air column decreases (this *increases* the column's resonant frequency), and higher frequency components of the "splashing" are emphasized. We know from experience that, when the pitch of the sound from the bottle is high enough, little air is left in the bottle and it is time to turn off the tap.

The simple spring-mass combination has only one resonant frequency; columns of air have many different resonant frequencies. We will consider only the resonances of tubes whose cross-sectional dimensions are small compared to the wavelengths of the sounds applied to them. The vocal tract is just this sort of tube for the frequencies of primary interest in speech.

A tube with uniform cross-sectional area throughout its

length has regularly spaced resonant frequencies. The values of these resonant frequencies depend on the length of the tube. Consider a tube closed at one end and open at the other. The lowest resonant frequency of this tube corresponds to the frequency of a sound wave whose length is four times the length of the tube. The value of the tube's other resonant frequencies will be odd-number multiples (three times, five times, etc.) of this lowest resonant frequency. When the cross-sectional area varies along the tube's length, the resonant frequencies are no longer uniformly spaced. They are spaced irregularly, some close together and some far apart, depending on the exact shape of the tube.

The human vocal tract is about 17 centimeters long and—at least when it produces vowel sounds—we can regard it as closed at one end and open at the other (the lips). The lowest resonant frequency of a uniform tube this long is 500 cps; its other resonant frequencies are 1500 cps, 2500 cps, 3500 cps, and so on.

When both ends of the tube are closed, the lowest resonant frequency is actually zero. The next resonant frequency, for a uniform tube, has a value corresponding to the frequency of a sound wave whose wavelength is twice as long as the tube. The values of the other resonant frequencies are even-numbered multiples of this next-to-lowest frequency.

As we will see in Chapter 4, the vocal tract is a tube of complicated shape that acts as a resonator. Its shape is varied by movements of the vocal organs. The resulting changes in its resonant frequencies play an important part in speech production.

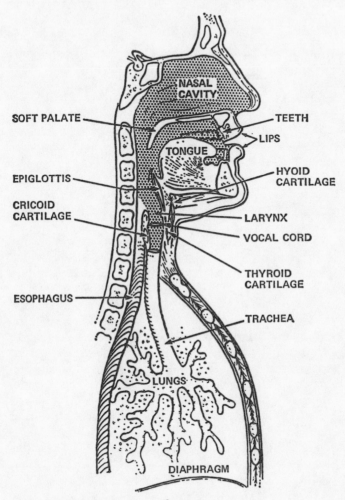

Fig. 17. The human vocal organs.

Chapter 4

SPEECH PRODUCTION

One of the important links in the speech chain is speech production, the specialized movements of our vocal organs that generate speech sound waves. Expressions like "his lips are sealed," "mother tongue" and "tongue-tied," are ample evidence that man has always understood the vital contribution of these organs to speech production.

The lips and tongue, however, are not the only organs associated with speech production. In this chapter, we shall describe all the organs involved; we shall explain how they function during speech and how the sound waves are produced.

The chapter has four sections. First, we have a quick look at the speech mechanism as a whole. Next, we describe the vocal organs, one by one. In the third section, we explain how these organs move to produce each English speech sound. The last section is concerned with the acoustics (or physics) of how the vocal organs produce and shape the sound waves of speech.

A BRIEF DESCRIPTION
OF SPEECH PRODUCTION

A diagram of the *vocal organs,* those parts of the body connected with speech production, is given in Fig. 17. The vocal organs are the *lungs,* the *windpipe,* the *larynx,* (containing the *vocal cords*), the throat or *pharynx,* the *nose* and the *mouth.* Together, these organs form an intricately shaped "tube" extending from the lungs to the lips. One part of the tube, lying above the larynx, is called the *vocal tract,* and consists of the pharynx, mouth and nose. The shape of the vocal tract can be varied extensively by moving the tongue, the lips and other parts of the tract.

The source of energy for speech production is the steady stream of air that comes from the lungs as we exhale. When we breathe normally, the air stream is inaudible. It can be made audible by setting it into rapid vibration. This can happen unintentionally; when we snore, for example. During speech, of course, we intentionally set the air stream into vibration. We can do this several ways, but the method most frequently used is by vocal cord action.

The vocal cords are part of the larynx. They constitute an adjustable barrier across the air passage coming from the lungs. When the vocal cords are open, the air stream passes into the vocal tract; when closed, they shut off the air flow from the lungs. As we talk, the vocal cords open and close rapidly, chopping up the steady air stream into a series of puffs. We can hear this rapid sequence of puffs as a buzz whose frequency gets higher and higher as we increase the vibration rate of the vocal cords. The character of the vocal cord buzz is modified by the vocal tract's acoustic properties. These acoustic properties depend on the shape of the vocal tract. During speech, we continually alter this shape by moving the tongue and the lips, etc. These movements, by altering the acoustic properties of the vocal tract, enable us to produce the different sounds of speech.

Adjusting the vocal tract's shape to produce different speech sounds is called *articulation*; the individual movements of the tongue, lips and other parts of the vocal tract are called articulatory movements.

We see, then, that air flow from the lungs provides the energy for speech wave production, that the vocal cords convert this energy into an audible buzz and that the tongue, lips, palate, etc.—by altering the shape of the vocal tract—transform the buzz into distinguishable speech sounds.

The mechanism just described is used for producing most speech waves. Two other methods are available for making the air stream from the lungs audible. In one, the vocal tract is constricted at some point along its length. The air stream passing through the constriction becomes turbulent, just like steam escaping through the narrow nozzle of a boiling tea kettle. This turbulent air stream sounds like a hiss and is, in fact, the hissy or *fricative* noise we make when pronouncing sounds like "s" or "sh."

The other method is to stop the flow of air altogether —but only momentarily—by blocking the vocal tract with the tongue or the lips, and then suddenly releasing the air pressure built up behind this block. We use the "blocking" technique to make sounds like "p" and "g," which are called *plosives*. It should be remembered that the second and third methods described are independent of vocal cord activity, although the speaker can vibrate his vocal cords simultaneously. Whichever of the three techniques is used, the resonances of the vocal tract still modify the character of the basic sounds produced by hiss, plosion or vocal cord vibration.

We may mention a few other methods that can be used for speech production, even though their use is infrequent. Producing a whisper is like making a hiss sound, except that the constriction that agitates the air stream is provided by holding the vocal cords still and close together. In some African languages, "clicks" are used. Clicks are produced by blocking the vocal tract at two points, sucking the air out from between the two blocks and then re-opening the tract. Some foreign languages use sounds produced while inhaling, but English speech is normally produced only while exhaling.

THE VOCAL ORGANS

We can now consider the action of the vocal organs in more detail. You may be interested to know, incidentally, that the primary biological function of the vocal organs is not speech production. They developed first to perform other vital services, such as breathing, chewing and swallowing. Only later were they applied to the production of speech.

The lungs are masses of spongy, elastic material in the rib cage. They supply oxygen to the blood and dispose of certain waste products like carbon dioxide. The act of breathing air in and out is controlled by various muscles of the rib cage, and by muscles of the abdomen and the diaphragm, the partition that separates the chest from the abdomen. During speech, the diaphragm relaxes and the degree of abdominal muscle contraction controls the extent to which the contents of the abdomen are pressed up against the diaphragm and carried into the chest cavity, where they squeeze air out of the lungs.

Normally, the lungs contain about three quarts of air. In addition, we regularly breathe in and out about one-half quart of air. If we first inhale deeply and then breathe out as far as we can, we may exhale as much as three and a half quarts of air, leaving about one and a half quarts of residual air in the lungs.

When we exhale, the air pressure from the lungs is only slightly above atmospheric pressure. It is about one-quarter of one per cent greater than atmospheric pressure when we breathe normally, and approximately one per cent greater than atmospheric during conversation.

Normally, we breathe about once every five seconds; roughly equal parts of this period are devoted to exhaling and inhaling. During speech, we can influence our breathing rate in accordance with the needs of sentence and phrase length; since we talk only while exhaling, we can adjust this rate to devote as little as 15 per cent of the breathing cycle to inhaling.

Air from the lungs travels up the *trachea* (see Fig. 17), a tube consisting of rings of cartilage, and through the larynx toward the mouth and nose.

The larynx acts as a gate or valve between the lungs and the mouth. By opening or closing, it controls the flow of air from the lungs; when it is shut tightly, it completely isolates the lungs from the mouth. Because the larynx can close the air passages, it plays an essential part in speech production, and in eating and breathing.

We take in both food and air through the mouth. When these essential commodities reach the back of the mouth—the pharynx—they face two downward openings: the larynx, leading through the trachea to the lungs, and the food pipe or *esophagus*, leading to the stomach (see Fig. 17). Food and air should not enter the wrong passage if our body is to function properly. We all know how unpleasant it is when food or any foreign matter finds its way into our windpipe—goes "down the wrong place," in other words. The larynx prevents this by closing automatically during swallowing to exclude food from the trachea and lungs.

Another function of the laryngeal valve is to lock air into the lungs. Animals which use their forelimbs extensively—especially tree climbing mammals—have a well developed larynx, because the arms can exert greater force when they are given rigid support by the air locked in the chest cavity. You can try this yourself. See how much the power of your arms is weakened if you fail to hold your breath. Normally, we unconsciously hold our breath when we do heavy work with our arms.

Man has learned to use his laryngeal valve to convert the steady air stream from the lungs into audible sound. He uses his larynx to break the air flow into a series of puffs, which is heard as a buzz; it is the sound wave we use in speech.

Constructionally, the larynx is a stack of cartilages. You can locate your larynx easily because one of its cartilages, the thyroid, is the projection on your neck known as the Adam's apple. Fig. 18 shows various views of the larynx's principal cartilages. The cartilages and their connecting muscles and ligaments form a series of rings about three inches high and less than two inches across. The larynx is not held in one rigid position; it can move up and down during swallowing and speaking.

At the top of the larynx is the pear-shaped *epiglottis*. Its narrow end is attached to the Adam's apple and its other end is free. During swallowing, the epiglottis helps to deflect food away from the windpipe, performing part of the larynx's valve function.

The valve action of the larynx depends largely on the *vocal cords*. The vocal cords are folds of ligament that extend, one on either side of the larynx, from the Adam's

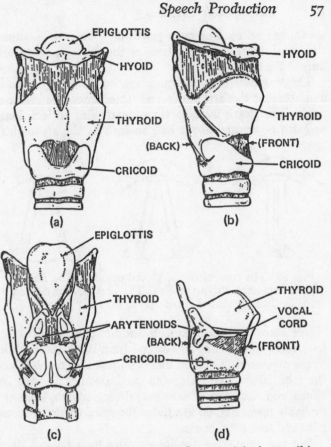

Fig. 18. Various views of the larynx: (a) front; (b) side; (c) back; (d) cutaway side.

apple at the front to the *arytenoid* cartilages at the back. The space between the vocal cords is called the *glottis*. When the arytenoids—and, therefore, the vocal cords— are pressed together, the air passage is completely sealed off and the laryngeal valve is shut. The glottal opening can be controlled by moving the arytenoids apart, as shown in Fig. 19. The open glottis is "V-shaped," because the vocal cords, held together at the front, move apart only at the back.

The length of the vocal cords can be altered by moving and rotating the arytenoids and, sometimes, the Adam's apple. The glottis is about three quarters of an inch long and can be opened about half an inch by the arytenoids.

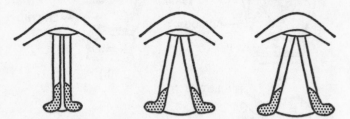

Fig. 19. The control of the glottal opening. The shaded areas represent the arytenoids. The curved, top portion of the figure is the Adam's apple.

Just above the vocal cords is another pair of folds, the *false vocal cords*. They also extend from the Adam's apple to the arytenoids. Opinion differs on just how much effect the false cords have on speech production. They can be closed and they can vibrate but, during speech, they are probably open. Fig. 20 illustrates the relationship between false and true vocal cords.

We see, then, that the larynx provides a triple barrier across the windpipe through the action of the epiglottis, the false vocal cords and the true vocal folds. All three are closed during swallowing and wide open during normal breathing.

What does the larynx do during speech? When we talk, the epiglottis and false vocal cords remain open, but the vocal cords close. Air pressure builds up behind the vocal cord barrier and eventually blows the cords apart. Once

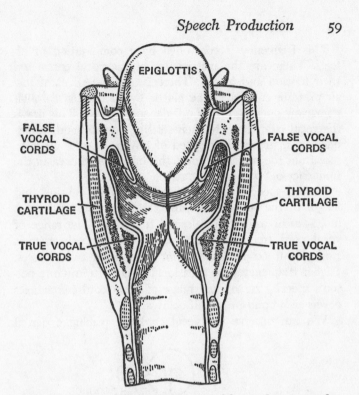

Fig. 20. The relationship between false and true vocal cords.

apart, the excess pressure is released, the cords return to their closed position, the pressure builds up again and the cycle repeats. The vibrating vocal cords rhythmically open and close the air passage between the lungs and mouth. They interrupt the steady air flow and produce the sequence of air puffs mentioned earlier. The frequency of vocal cord vibration and, consequently, the frequency of the air puffs, is determined by how fast the cords are blown apart and how fast they snap back into their closed position.

This frequency is controlled by a combination of effects. There are the massiveness of the vocal cords and their tension and length. There is also the effect of low air pressure created in the glottis by air rushing through its narrow opening into the wider space above. This draws the vocal cords back to their starting position and, consequently, increases their speed of return. Greater air pressure from the lungs enhances this effect and increases the frequency of vocal cord vibration.

During speech, we continually alter the tension and length of the vocal cords—and the air pressure from the lungs—until we get the desired frequency. The range of vocal cord frequencies used in normal speech extends from about 60 to 350 cps, or more than two octaves. Higher frequencies are occasionally used. In any one person's speech, the normal range of vocal cord frequencies covers about one and a half octaves.

We can observe the vocal cords by placing a dental

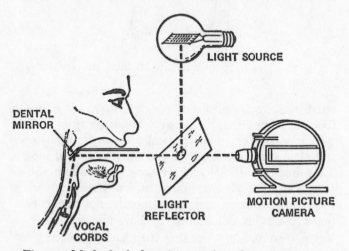

Fig. 21. Method of observing vocal cord movement.

mirror in a speaker's mouth, as shown in Fig. 21. The vocal cords vibrate so rapidly, however, that their movements are not clear when observed this way. We can see much more by filming what appears in the dental mirror with a special high-speed camera, and viewing the film in slow motion. Observations of this kind show that the vibrating vocal cords move up and down as well as sideways, although the sideways movement predominates. The slow motion films also show that the vocal cords do not always close completely during their vibration cycle.

Suitable measurements have enabled us to determine how the air puffs vary throughout the glottal cycle. Fig.

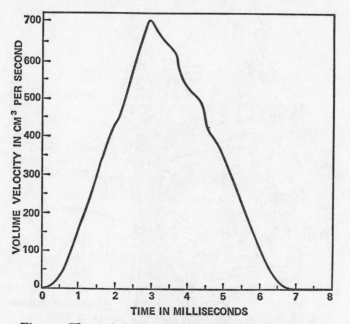

Fig. 22. The variation of air flow in a glottal puff. The curve repeats once every 8 milliseconds (a frequency of 125 cps).

22 shows a typical curve. The spectrum of such pressure waves has many components, but their frequencies are always whole-number multiples of the vocal cord frequency. Their amplitudes generally decrease as their frequency increases. In loud speech and shouting, the vocal cords open and close more rapidly and remain open for a smaller fraction of a cycle; this increases the amplitude of the higher harmonics and gives the sounds a harsher quality.

We have seen how the energy for speech is provided by the air stream from the lungs and how vocal cord vi-

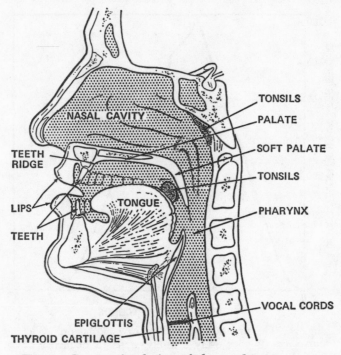

Fig. 23. Cross-sectional view of the vocal tract.

bration generates an audible buzz. Let us go on to see how the quality of this buzz is changed by the configuration of the vocal tract. A cross-sectional view of the vocal tract is shown in Fig. 23. The vocal tract extends from the glottis to the lips—by way of the pharynx and mouth—with a side branch into the nasal passages.

The *pharynx* is the part of the vocal tract nearest the glottis. It is a tube connecting the larynx with the mouth and the nose. At its lower end, the pharynx meets the larynx and the esophagus and, at its wider upper end, joins with the back of the mouth and the nose, as shown in Fig. 24. We have known for some time that its shape and size are changed when swallowing, either by moving the tongue back, or the larynx up, or by contracting the pharyngeal walls. Only recently, however, has it been noticed that such changes take place during speech. These changes can be seen clearly in the vocal tract outlines shown in Fig. 25. Very little is known about the pharyngeal changes we make for distinguishing one speech sound from another. As a result, we shall not have much to say about the pharynx later in this chapter, when we describe the movements of the vocal organs for articulating English speech sounds.

The nasal cavity (see Fig. 23), extending from the pharynx to the nostrils, is about four inches long. It is divided into two sections by the *septum,* a central partition that runs along the entire length of the cavity. Ridges and folds in the cavity's walls break up some segments of the nasal air passages into intricately shaped channels. At the back of the nose—and also lower down in the pharynx —are the *tonsils* (see Fig. 23). They occasionally grow large enough to influence the air flow from the lungs and, when they do, they add the characteristic "adenoidal" quality to the voice. The sensory endings of the nerve

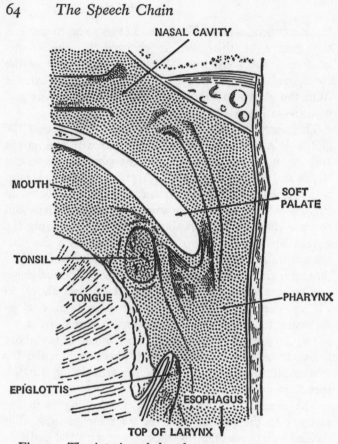

Fig. 24. The interior of the pharynx.

concerned with smell are also located in the nose. The nasal cavities can be isolated from the pharynx and the back of the mouth by raising the *soft palate* (to be described in a later section of this chapter).

The last and most important part of the vocal tract is the mouth. Its shape and size can be varied—more extensively than any other part of the vocal tract—by adjust-

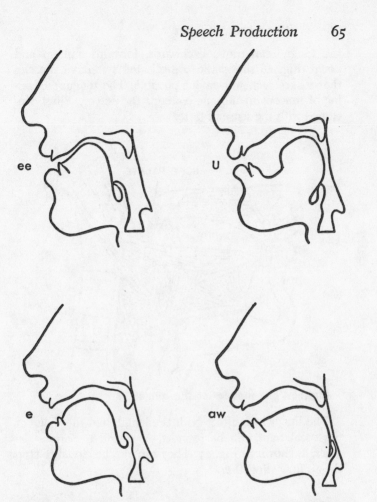

Fig. 25. Outlines of the vocal tract during the articulation of various vowels.

ing the relative positions of the palate, the tongue, the lips and the teeth.

The most flexible of these is the tongue. Its tip, its edges and its center can be moved independently; the entire tongue can move backwards, forwards and up and down. Fig. 26 shows the complicated system of muscles that makes such movement possible. The tongue's covering of mucous membrane contains the nerve endings concerned with the sense of taste.

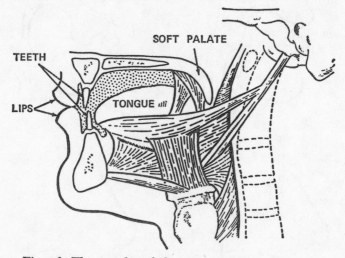

Fig. 26. The muscles of the tongue.

The lips, which affect both the length and the shape of the vocal tract, can be rounded or spread to various degrees, as shown in Fig. 27. They can also be closed to stop the air flow altogether.

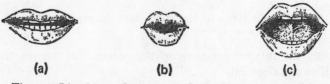

(a)   (b)   (c)

Fig. 27. Lip shapes during articulation: (a) spread; (b) rounded; (c) unrounded.

The lips and the cheeks influence speech communication in more than one way. They change the shape of the vocal tract and, consequently, the kind of speech sound produced. But, together with the teeth, they are the only parts of the vocal tract normally visible. The listener can gather information about what the speaker is saying by watching his face as well as listening to his voice. This is called *lip reading*, and it has a more significant effect on speech communication than most people give it credit for. If you have ever had a conversation in really noisy surroundings, you know how useful it is to see the speaker's face. Most deaf people can understand some of what you say just by watching your face.

There is still another way the lips and cheeks play a part in speech communication. Their shape contributes to setting the facial expressions that give an indication of your emotions; this can help a listener understand speech that might otherwise be insufficiently intelligible.

The teeth also affect the vocal tract's shape and the sounds it produces. They can be used to restrict or stop the air flow by placing them close to the lips or the tip of the tongue, as in the sounds "v" or "th," for example.

The last of the organs that shape the mouth cavity is the *palate*. We can divide it into three parts. They are the teeth ridge or *alveolus*, covered by the gums; the bony *hard palate* that forms the roof of the mouth; and the muscular *soft palate* at the back. If you stand in front of a mirror and open your mouth wide, you will see your soft palate moving up and down at the back of your mouth. The soft palate is normally lowered, taking up roughly the position shown in Fig. 23. It can be raised, however, and in this position it closes the opening between the pharynx and the nose (see Fig. 28), and the air expelled from the lungs is directed entirely along the mouth.

This completes our description of all the organs im-

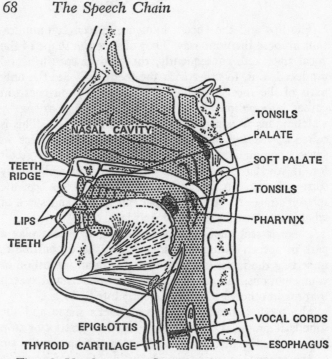

Fig. 28. Vocal tract configuration for articulating non-nasal sounds.

portant in shaping the vocal tract. By setting the shape of the vocal tract—and its acoustic characteristics—the vocal organs enable us to distinguish one speech sound from another. Let us see, now, how these organs move in articulating the sounds of spoken English.

THE ARTICULATION OF ENGLISH SPEECH SOUNDS

For convenience, we will divide the speech sounds into two groups, vowels and consonants.

The vocal cords vibrate during the articulation of vowels; they also vibrate when making some of the consonants. Sounds produced with vocal cord vibration are called *voiced*. Sounds produced without vocal cord vibration are called *unvoiced*.

We will describe the articulation of vowels in terms of tongue and lip positions. Some speakers raise their soft palates during vowel production, shutting off the nasal cavities, while others leave it partially lowered. The added nasal quality is not used to distinguish one English vowel from another.

It is not so easy to describe the positions of the tongue. The tongue is highly mobile and its tip, edges and main body can move independently. Experience has shown that its configuration can best be described by specifying where the main body of the tongue is. The position of the highest part of the main body is called the *position of the tongue*.

The tongue positions used for making vowels are usually described by comparing them with the positions used for making a number of references of *cardinal vowels*. The cardinal vowels are a set of standard reference sounds whose quality is defined independently of any language. They form a yardstick of vowel quality against which the quality of any other vowel can be measured. The cardinal vowel system is basically a system of perceptual qualities, but X-ray experiments show substantial agreement between vowel quality and tongue position. It has become acceptable, therefore, to compare the tongue positions of vowels with those of the cardinal vowels. Strictly speaking, no written definition of cardinal vowel quality is possible because the "definition" of quality is perceived only when listening to a trained phonetician making the sounds. However, we may hazard an approximate definition. When a person moves his tongue as high up and as far forward as he can—without narrowing the width of the air passage to produce a hiss—and spreads his lips at the same time, an "ee"-like sound is produced. If he now keeps the tongue high, moves it back as far as he can and rounds his lips, he will make an "oo" sound. If the tongue is moved down as far as possible, still keeping it far back, and the lips are unrounded, he produces a sound very much like the "o" in the word "long." These are three of the cardinal vowels.

By mapping the tongue positions for these three, we get the diagram shown in Fig. 29(a). The other five cardinal vowels are defined as those sounds that divide the

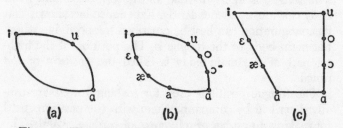

(a)   (b)   (c)

Fig. 29. Tongue positions for cardinal vowel articulation: (a) cardinal vowels 1, 5, and 8; (b) the eight cardinal vowels; (c) schematic representation of tongue positions for the same eight cardinal vowels as in (b).

distances between the three mapped positions into perceptually equal sections. Fig. 29(b) shows a map of the corresponding tongue positions and (c) the conventional form in which the tongue positions of (b) are usually shown. Fig. 29(c) is the so-called *vowel quadrilateral*. All the tongue positions of the cardinal vowels are along the outer limits of tongue movement. If the position of the tongue moves toward the center of the mouth, the quality of the sound becomes more neutral and "uh"-like.

When the tongue is near the palate, the sound produced is called a *close* vowel; when the tongue is low, at the bottom of the mouth, the vowel is called *open*. Sounds produced with the tongue near the center of the vowel quadrilateral are called *central* or *neutral* vowels. The sound "ee," therefore, is a *close front* vowel, and "oo" a *close back* vowel; "ah" and "aw" are *open front* and *open back* vowels, respectively.

Basically, any lip configuration could be used with any tongue position. In English, however, front vowels are usually made with spread lips and back vowels with rounded lips; as the tongue is lowered to more open positions, the lips tend to become unrounded. Native speakers of English find it difficult to go against this "rule," and some of us might even say that the muscles of our mouths are so constructed that these lip shapes and tongue positions must necessarily go together. This is really only a matter of habit, however. Other languages do have sounds with a different relationship between lips and tongue.

In Russian, for example, there is a vowel made with the tongue in a close back position (as for the English "oo"), but with the lips parted (as for the English "ee"). Again, in French, there is a vowel made with the tongue in a close front position (as for the English "ee"), but with the lips rounded (as for the English "oo").

Why not try to make this French vowel? It is that elusive sound used in "rue," the French word for "street." At first, you might find it impossible, but if you persist, perhaps even using your fingers to round your lips, while keeping your tongue in the position for an English "ee," you will no doubt succeed.

Let us return to English sounds. Fig. 30 shows the tongue positions for the principal English vowels. The vowels shown in this figure are the so-called *pure* vowels, which means that their quality remains substantially unchanged

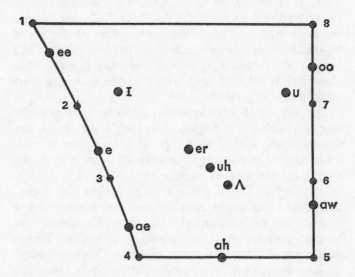

THE PURE VOWELS

ee	heat	ah	father
I	hit	aw	call
e	head	U	put
ae	had	oo	cool
uh	the	ʌ	ton
	er	bird	

THE DIPHTHONGS

ou	tone
ei	take
ai	might
au	shout
oi	toil

Fig. 30. Tongue positions for English vowels (the tongue positions for the eight cardinal vowels are shown by numerals).

throughout the syllables in which they are used. There is another group of English vowels, the *diphthongs* (pronounced, "dif-thongs"); the diphthong is a sound whose quality changes noticeably from its beginning to its end in a syllable. The principle diphthongs of English are also listed in Fig. 30. The tongue movements associated with these sounds are roughly movements between positions assumed for pure vowels. For the diphthong "au," for example, the tongue would move roughly from the position for the sound "ah" to the position for the sound "ʊ" and so forth.

The English consonants are best described by specifying their *place-of-articulation* and their *manner-of-articulation*; they are further distinguished by whether they are voiced or unvoiced.

The significant places-of-articulation in English are the lips, the teeth, the gums, the palate and the glottis. The categories of manner-of-articulation are *plosive, fricative, nasal, liquid* and *semi-vowel*.

The plosive consonants, for example, are made by blocking the air pressure somewhere along the mouth and then suddenly releasing the pressure. The airflow can be blocked by pressing the lips together or by pressing the tongue against either the gums or the soft palate. We can have plosives, then, with a *labial* (lips), *alveolar* (gums) or *velar* (soft palate) place-of-articulation.

Similarly, fricatives are made by constricting the air flow somewhere in the mouth—enough to make the air turbulent—to produce sound of a hissy quality. The fricatives, like the plosives, differ according to their places-of-articulation. The nasals are made by lowering the soft palate, coupling the nasal cavities to the pharynx, and blocking the mouth somewhere along its length to produce different places-of-articulation. All other English consonants are made with the soft palate raised.

The English semi-vowels are the "w" and "y" sounds. Both are produced by keeping the vocal tract briefly in a vowel-like position, and then changing it rapidly to the position required for the following vowel in the syllable. Consequently, the semi-vowels must always be followed by a vowel in whatever syllable they are used. The consonant "y" is formed by putting the tongue in the close frontal position required for an "ee" sound, holding it there briefly and then changing to whatever vowel follows the "y." Forming the "w" is similar, except that the lips are first close rounded, as required for an "oo." "W" and "y," therefore, have a labial and alveolar place-of-articulation, respectively. They are both voiced consonants.

The only English lateral consonant is "l." It is made by putting the tip of the tongue against the gums and allowing the air to pass on either side of the tongue. It is a voiced consonant.

A classification of all English consonants, according to place- and manner-of-articulation, is given in Table V.

TABLE V—CLASSIFICATION OF ENGLISH CONSONANTS BY
PLACE- AND MANNER-OF-ARTICULATION

Place of articulation	Manner of articulation				
	Plosive	Fricative	Semi-vowel	Liquids (incl. laterals)	Nasal
Labial	p b		w		m
Labio-Dental		f v			
Dental		θ th			
Alveolar	t d	s z	y	l r	n
Palatal		sh zh			
Velar	k g				ng
Glottal		h			

The vocal tract configurations we have described are not, of course, made exactly this way every time a speech sound is produced. We have described typical (idealized) articulations and considerable deviations from these occur in actual speech. Deviations can be due to the individual habits of different speakers. They can also occur because of the influence of other sounds that immediately precede or follow the sound being uttered. For example, the sound "k" is made by pressing the back of the tongue against the soft palate. Just where the tongue and palate meet depends a lot on what the following vowel is; if it is a back vowel, like an "oo," the contact will be much further back than with an "ee." Again, in fast speech, we often start the articulation of a particular sound—that is, move the tongue or lips toward the specified position—without finishing the movement before going on to the next sound. Despite all these variations, speech is still intelligible. Why this is so will be discussed in later chapters.

Now that we have seen how the movements of the various vocal organs shape the vocal tract tube, we can consider the tube's acoustic effect on the character of sounds produced.

THE ACOUSTICS OF SPEECH PRODUCTION

You will recall that the buzz-like sound produced by the vocal cords is applied to the vocal tract. The vocal tract is, in effect, an air-filled tube and, like all air-filled tubes, acts as a resonator. This means that the vocal tract has certain natural frequencies of vibration, and that it responds more readily to a sound wave whose frequency is the same as its resonant frequency than to a sound wave of another frequency. Let us assume, for example, that the vocal cords produce a series of pulses as shown in Fig. 31(a). The spectrum of such a sound has a large number of components; all of them are more or less of the same amplitude and have frequencies that are whole-number multiples of the fundamental frequency. The fundamental—the spectrum's lowest frequency component—has the same frequency as the vocal cords' frequency of vibration. When such a wave is applied at one end of the vocal tract (at the glottis), and is transmitted towards the lips, the vocal tract responds better to those components of the vocal cord puffs that are at or near its natural frequency. These components will be emphasized and the spectrum of the sound emerging from the lips will "peak" at the natural frequency of the vocal tract. This is the process illustrated in Fig. 31. Fig. 31(b) shows the spectrum of the vocal cord output and (c) shows the frequency response of a simple resonator; (d) and (e) are the waveshape and spectrum of the sound wave produced when the sound of (a) is transmitted through the resonator of (c).

The resonator of Fig. 31(c) has only one natural frequency, but the vocal tract has many. The vocal resonator, therefore, will emphasize the harmonics of the vocal cord wave at a number of different frequencies, and the spectrum of the speech wave will have a peak for each of the vocal tract's natural frequencies. The values of the natural frequencies of the vocal tract are determined by its shape; consequently, the amplitudes of the spectral components will peak at different frequencies as we change the shape of the tract. Fig. 32 shows the spectra of sounds produced for three different vocal tract shapes.

Resonances of the vocal tract are called *formants,* and their frequencies, the *formant frequencies.* Every configuration of the vocal tract has its own set of characteristic formant frequencies.

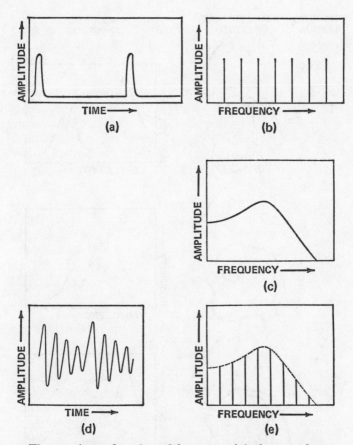

Fig. 31. An explanation of formants: (a) the waveshape
of a pulse train; (b) a spectrum of a train of short pulses;
(c) frequency response of a simple resonator; (d) and
(e) are the waveshape and the spectrum, respectively,
of a sound wave produced when a series of pulses, like
those of (a), is applied to a resonator whose frequency
response is shown in (c).

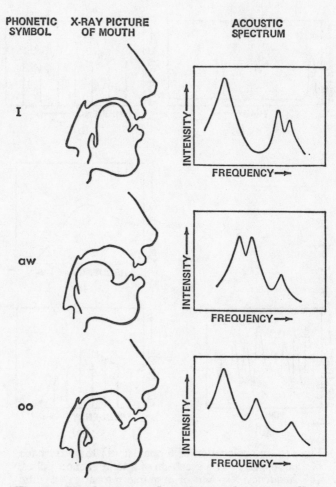

Fig. 32. Vocal tract configurations and corresponding spectra for three different vowels. (The peaks of the spectra represent vocal tract resonances. Vertical lines for individual harmonics are not shown.)

You may have noticed in Fig. 31 that the resonant frequency is not equal to the frequency of any harmonic of the spectrum. In general, the frequencies of the formants will not be the same as those of the harmonics, although they may coincide. After all, there is no reason why they should agree. The formant frequencies are determined by the vocal tract, the harmonic frequencies by the vocal cords, and the vocal tract and vocal cords can move independently of each other. The independence of vocal cord and formant frequencies is shown in Figs. 33 and 34. Fig.

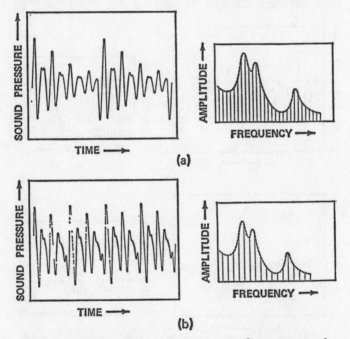

Fig. 33. The waveshapes and corresponding spectra of the vowel "ah" pronounced with two different vocal cord frequencies: (a) vocal cord frequency equals 90 cps; (b) vocal cord frequency equals 150 cps.

33 (a) shows the waveshape and spectrum of the sound "ah" produced with the vocal cords vibrating at 90 cps; (b) shows the waveshape and spectrum of the same sound with the cords vibrating at 150 cps. Even though the frequencies of all the harmonics have changed, the frequencies of the formants (and of the spectral peaks) are unaltered because the shape of the vocal tract remained the same. In Fig. 34(a), we again see the waveshape and spectrum of the sound "ah" at 90 cps; in (b), the vocal cord vibration is still 90 cps, but the shape of the vocal tract has been changed to produce the sound "uh." In

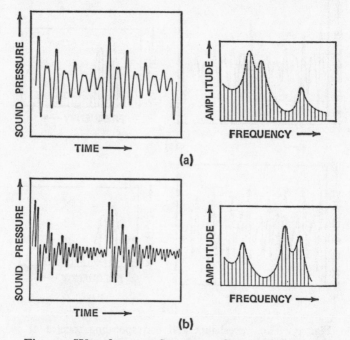

Fig. 34. Waveshapes and corresponding spectra of the vowels "ah" and "uh" pronounced with a vocal cord frequency of 90 cps: (a) "ah"; (b) "uh."

Fig. 34(a) and (b), the frequency of vocal cord vibration and, therefore, the frequencies of the harmonics, are the same; the shape of the vocal tract is changed, however, with a corresponding change in the position of the formants (and of the spectral peaks). The figures clearly show that the vocal tract does not affect the frequency of the harmonics, but simply emphasizes the amplitudes of those harmonics that happen to be similar to its own natural, resonant frequency.

Unfortunately, the sound spectra produced by the vocal cords are not always as regular as the one shown in Fig. 31(b). The vocal cord spectrum may have its own peaks and valleys; the vocal tract formants will just add more irregularities. The speech spectrum, then, may well have peaks that were not produced by vocal tract resonances. In transmitting speech waves, it would often be useful to know the formant frequencies, and one of the troublesome—and important—problems of present-day speech research is to find ways of determining which of the speech spectrum's numerous peaks are produced by formants and which are due to other causes.

In the previous chapter, resonance was explained in two different ways. First, as a characteristic of oscillating systems—pendulums, springs and air-filled tubes—when exposed to vibratory forces of different frequencies. We saw that such systems respond more readily to excitation frequencies near their natural frequency. Second, we saw that when a resonator is disturbed and then left alone, it will continue to vibrate at its own natural frequency. Of course, these descriptions are just two different views of the same event. Similarly, there are two different ways to explain the effect of the vocal tract resonances on speech production. So far, we have taken the view that a resonator will respond more readily to excitation at or near its own natural frequency. We could also take the view that each time a puff of air "hits" the vocal tract resonator, the vocal tract continues to "ring" at its own natural frequency. In the simple resonator of Fig. 31(c), every air puff from the vocal cords will generate sinusoidal oscillation at the resonator's natural frequency; the oscillation will decay at a rate determined by its damping. This is shown in Fig. 31(d). The spectrum of such a train of damped sinusoids is the spectrum already discussed and shown in Fig. 31(e). The vocal tract has many resonant frequencies. It will "ring" at all its natural frequencies simultaneously, and the vibration resulting from the impact of each air puff will now be the sum of a number of damped sinusoids. Fig. 35(a) shows the waveshape of the sound "ah" and how the same oscillation repeats for every puff of vocal cord sound. Fig. 35(b) shows the spectrum of such a wave train. It is identical to the spectrum of "ah" in Fig. 33(a), and we can again see that our explanations represent two views of the same event.

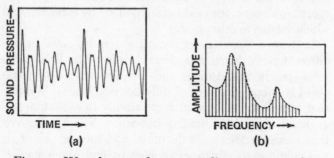

Fig. 35. Waveshape and corresponding spectrum of a vowel sound: (a) the waveshape; (b) the spectrum.

Formant frequency values depend on the shape of the vocal tract. When the soft palate is raised, shutting off the nasal cavities, the vocal tract is a tube about seven inches long from the glottis to the lips. For such a tube (with a uniform cross-sectional area along its whole length), the principal resonances will be at 500 cps, 1500 cps, 2500 cps, 3500 cps and 4500 cps. In general, the cross-sectional area of the vocal tract varies considerably along its length. As a result, its formant frequencies will not be as regularly spaced as for a uniform tube; some of them will be higher in frequency and others lower. The lowest formant frequency is called the *first formant*; the one with the next highest frequency, the *second formant*, and so forth.

When the soft palate is lowered—coupling the nasal cavities to the mouth—a basically different vocal tract shape is formed. The vocal tract starts as a single tube in the pharynx, but separates into two branches at the soft palate, one through the nose and the other through the mouth. We now have different formants because of the additional nasal branch, and we have anti-resonances that suppress parts of the speech spectrum. The nasal cavities also absorb more sound energy; this will increase the damping and reduce the amplitudes of the formants. The speech wave produced depends greatly on whether and where the mouth cavity is obstructed, as in other speech sounds.

Much more research has to be done before we can fully explain how the characteristics of the sounds produced depend on the shape of the vocal tract. Even where the process is fairly well understood, complicated mathematics is needed for the calculation of the formants. As a result, much of what we know about the formants of speech sounds is obtained simply by examining the sounds produced when the vocal tract has a given shape, rather than by explaining how these formants came about. Examination of the acoustic characteristics of speech waves has not only produced more information about formants, but has brought to light other important features of speech waves. These results will be described in Chapter 7.

Chapter 5

HEARING

We accept with little question the immense variety of sensations to which we are exposed during daily life. The objects we see, the sounds we hear and the odors we smell obviously have some existence in the world around us. A little reflection makes it clear, however, that our internal image of the external world is produced by highly selective mechanisms. For example, the radio waves and gamma rays that pass through our bodies and the high frequency sounds of bats in flight are just as real as the familiar sound of a ringing telephone, the sight of trees and the feel of typewriter keys beneath the fingers. But activities outside the range of our senses pass unnoticed and unperceived. It is not until we lose some of our sensory capabilities that we realize how remarkable they are and how little of the "real" world exists for us without them.

For lower animals, the ability to hear can mean the difference between life and death. Locating prey is almost impossible for a deaf wolf. Even the proverbial early bird relies primarily on his sense of hearing to get his worm. In man, of course, hearing plays a vital role in the sequence of activities we have been calling *the speech chain.*

Regardless of the animal we consider, the physical function of the hearing sense organs is to receive acoustic vibrations and convert them into signals suitable for transmission along the auditory nerve toward the brain. Complex processing of these signals in the brain creates the perceptual world of sound.

In this chapter, we will consider two aspects of hearing. The first is the anatomy and physiology of the hearing organs, from the external portions of the ear to the point where sound stimuli are transformed into nervous activity. (The transmission of this activity to the brain and its processing there are discussed in Chapter 6.) This might be called the *sound reception* aspect of hearing.

The second aspect concerns *sound perception*; that is, the sensations we experience when exposed to different types of sound stimuli. Essentially, this area is the province of experimental psychology.

THE HEARING ORGANS

The Outer Ear   When examining the action of the ear, it is convenient to consider separately the outer, middle and inner ears, shown in Fig. 36. The outer ear, consisting of the externally visible portions of the ear and the ear canal, plays a relatively minor role in the hearing process. The *ear canal* is an air-filled passageway, about an inch long, closed at one end by the *eardrum* and open at the other end to the outside. Acoustic waves falling on the external ear funnel down the ear canal and set the eardrum into vibration. Because the ear canal is an acoustic *resonator* (see Chapter 3), it amplifies sound waves at frequencies near its resonant frequency. Thus, the pressure at the eardrum for tones near this resonance (about 3000 to 4000 cps) may be two to four times greater than the pressure at the entrance to the ear canal. This effect enables us to detect sounds that would be imperceptible if the eardrum were located at the surface of the head. Its position inside the head also serves to protect the sensitive eardrum from physical damage, and to make the temperature and humidity in its vicinity relatively independent of external conditions.

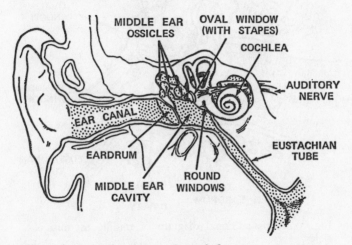

Fig. 36. Over-all cutaway view of the ear.

The Middle Ear The *middle ear* contains the *auditory ossicles,* three small bones (the malleus, the incus and the stapes) that form a mechanical linkage between the eardrum and the inner ear. The middle ear chamber is actually a cavity in the bones of the skull, as shown in Fig. 37. The ossicles are suspended within the cavity by several ligaments attached to the cavity walls. The handle of the *malleus* (hammer) is rigidly attached to the eardrum and covers more than one-half the drum area. Motions of the eardrum are transmitted by the malleus to the *incus* (anvil) which, in turn, is connected to the *stapes* (stirrup). The footplate of the stapes covers the *oval window,* which is the entrance to the inner ear.

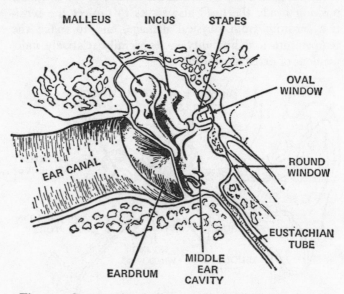

Fig. 37. Cross-sectional diagram of middle ear and ossicles.

If the middle ear cavity were completely sealed off from the outside air, the pressures inside and outside the cavity would generally differ. Forces exerted on the eardrum because of this pressure difference would tend to deform it. The *Eustachian tube,* running between the middle ear and mouth cavities, effectively links the middle ear with the outside air. The Eustachian tube is normally closed, and pressure differences can build up between the middle ear and the surrounding air. This is particularly noticeable if the outside air pressure changes fairly rapidly—as when rising in a fast elevator, taking off or landing in an airplane, or diving deep below the surface of a swimming pool. A small pressure difference usually results in slight discomfort, but large differences can lead to severe pain or even a ruptured eardrum. Swallowing normally causes the Eustachian tube to open momentarily, allowing the pressures to equalize.

The middle ear performs two major functions. First, it increases the amount of acoustic energy entering the fluid-filled inner ear. If a sound wave in air were to arrive at the oval window directly (for example, if the eardrum and ossicles were removed), almost all of the incident energy would be reflected, exactly as sound is reflected by any hard surface. To increase the efficiency with which sound energy is transmitted to the inner ear, it is necessary to increase the amplitude of the pressure variations at the oval window.

The middle ear accomplishes this amplification in two ways. First, as shown in Fig. 38(a), the ossicles behave like a lever mechanism, producing greater force at the stapes footplate than the force applied at the malleus. The ratio of these two forces is equal to the ratio of drum displacement to the displacement of the stapes. The increase is about a factor of 1.5. Second, and more important, the total force at the stapes is applied only over the area of the oval window, which is much smaller than the eardrum. The area of the eardrum is about 25 times greater than the area of the oval window, as shown schematically in Fig. 38(b). These effects combine to make the pressure at the oval window about 35 times greater than it would be if the eardrum and ossicles were not present. This pressure amplification in the middle ear en-

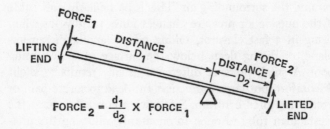

$$FORCE_2 = \frac{d_1}{d_2} \times FORCE_1$$

(a)

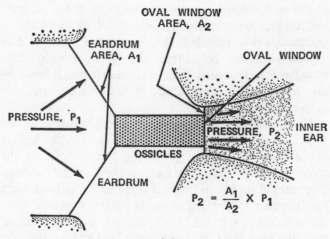

$$P_2 = \frac{A_1}{A_2} \times P_1$$

(b)

Fig. 38. The (a) portion shows the lever principle of the ossicles. The (b) portion is a diagrammatic representation of the area changing effect between the eardrum and oval window. The ossicles act as a piston pressing against the fluid of the inner ear.

ables us to hear sounds whose energies are about 1000 times weaker than we could hear otherwise.

The middle ear's second function is to protect the inner ear from extremely loud sounds. Several different actions are involved. Two small muscles, one connected to the eardrum and the other to the stapes, work in reflex response to loud sounds. One of them pulls in the drum, while the other draws the stapes away from the oval window. Both motions reduce the efficiency of the middle ear as a sound transmitter. Another protective mechanism changes the axis about which the stapes rotates. Ordinarily, the ossicles are suspended so that they vibrate as shown in Fig. 39(a). When the excitation becomes extremely severe, muscle contractions cause the ossicles to shift to a second mode of vibration, and the stapes moves as shown in (b). This substantially decreases the pressure variations transmitted to the inner ear, thus serving to protect its delicate structures. Unfortunately, neither of these protective mechanisms works instantaneously, and sudden, intense sounds can do permanent damage.

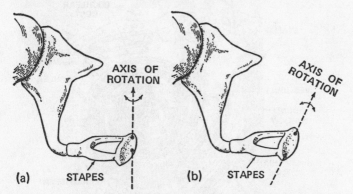

Fig. 39. Normal and high intensity modes of vibration of the stapes: (a) normal mode; (b) high intensity mode.

The Inner Ear   The *inner ear* is a small, intricate system of cavities in the bones of the skull. One cavity, coiled like a snail's shell, is called the *cochlea* (see Fig. 40). The important transformation from mechanical vibrations to nerve impulses takes place in the cochlea.

To see the parts of the cochlea more clearly, imagine that it could be unrolled as shown in Fig. 41(a). The cochlea is divided into two distinct regions along most of its length by a membranous structure called the *cochlear partition*. The interior of the partition forms a third region. On the oval window side of the cochlear partition is the *scala vestibuli*; the *scala tympani* lies on the other side. Both regions are filled with *perilymph,* a fluid almost twice as viscous as water. An opening in the cochlear partition at the apical end of the cochlea allows fluid to pass freely between the two cavities; the opening is called the *helicotrema.* At the basal end of the cochlea, the scala

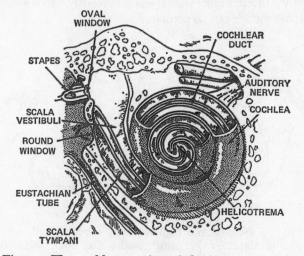

Fig. 40. The cochlear portion of the inner ear.

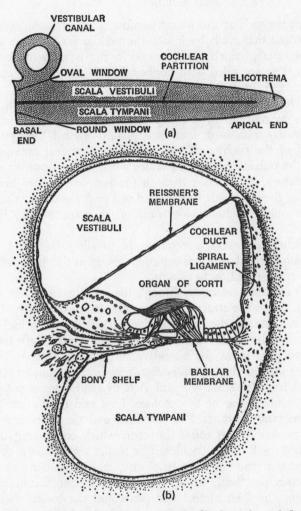

Fig. 41. Portion (a) shows a longitudinal section of the unrolled cochlea; portion (b) is a cross-section through the unrolled cochlea.

tympani ends at the *round window,* a membrane-covered opening that leads back into the middle ear. The vestibular canals, which play no role in the hearing mechanism, also are filled with perilymph, and are directly connected to the cochlea.

The cochlear structure is excited through the oval window by motions of the stapes footplate. When the window moves inward, fluid is displaced toward the apical end of the cochlea. If the motion is slow (for example, as the outside pressure increases when we go down in an elevator), fluid passes through the helicotrema and back along the other side to the basal end of the cochlea, where the round window moves outward to accommodate the flow.

Sound vibrations are too rapid to allow this kind of action; instead, pressure variations set up in the fluid cause the entire partition to vibrate.

A cross-section taken through the cochlea, as in Fig. 41 (b), shows the structure of the partition more clearly. Its hollow center, the *cochlear duct,* is filled with a highly viscous, almost jelly-like fluid called *endolymph. Reissner's Membrane* forms the boundary between the scala vestibuli and the duct; the *basilar membrane* separates the duct from the scala tympani. A bony shelf extends out of the central core of the cochlea. One end of the basilar membrane is attached to this shelf and the other end is connected to the *spiral ligament,* which coils along the outside wall of the cochlea. The basilar membrane is very narrow at the cochlea's basal end, where the bony shelf extends practically all the way across. Near the helicotrema, the shelf almost disappears and the basilar membrane occupies most of the space between the cochlear walls. There is a gradual transition between these extremes along the entire length of the cochlea. The basilar membrane, therefore, is actually narrowest at the basal end of the cochlea (about 0.04 millimeters wide), and widest (about 0.5 millimeters) at the apical end. Furthermore, it is quite stiff and light near the oval window, and most lax and massive near the helicotrema.

The mechanical properties of the basilar membrane are largely responsible for the way the cochlear partition responds to excitation through the oval window. If the stapes is suddenly displaced inward, say in response to a click, the cochlear partition first bulges downward—at the basal end—into the scala tympani. The bulge in the partition travels along the cochlea toward the helicotrema, broadening as it moves.

The response to sine-wave excitation is particularly revealing. The entire partition is set into vibration, but the amplitude of vibration at different points along the partition depends strongly on the applied frequency. For high frequencies, the vibration in the partition is highest near the oval window, where the basilar membrane is lightest and stiffest. For lower frequencies, the point of maximum amplitude moves toward the broader and more elastic end. The structure of the basilar membrane, then, leads to a spatial separation of the maximum response to stimulation at different frequencies. This action arises in much the same way that the long, heavy and relatively loose strings of a piano respond to low notes, while the short, light, taut strings vibrate in sympathy with high notes. At very low frequencies, say below 100 cps, the membrane vibrates as a whole, and the maximum amplitude occurs at the apical end.

Figure 42 shows displacement amplitudes along the cochlear partition for different frequencies of sine-wave excitation at the stapes. We should keep in mind that the partition goes through a considerably more complex motion than a simple up-and-down vibration between the curves shown in Fig. 42. For example, Fig. 43 shows the

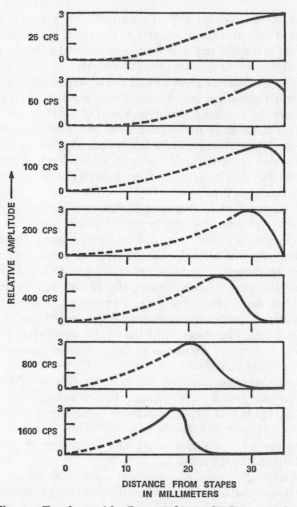

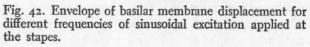

Fig. 42. Envelope of basilar membrane displacement for different frequencies of sinusoidal excitation applied at the stapes.

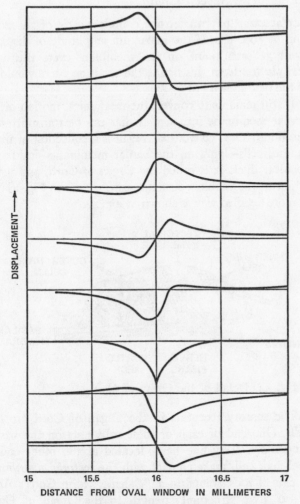

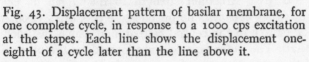

DISTANCE FROM OVAL WINDOW IN MILLIMETERS

Fig. 43. Displacement pattern of basilar membrane, for one complete cycle, in response to a 1000 cps excitation at the stapes. Each line shows the displacement one-eighth of a cycle later than the line above it.

displacement pattern for one complete cycle of an excitation of 1000 cps. If the maximum amplitude of displacement at each point on the membrane were measured and plotted from this figure, the resulting curve would be of the type shown in Fig. 42.

It still remains to convert the mechanical motion of the basilar membrane into signals that can be transmitted to the brain. The "converting" organ is a collection of many minute cells—lying on the basilar membrane—inside the cochlear duct. It is called the *Organ of Corti,* and its relation to the cochlear structure can be seen in Fig. 41(b). A more detailed view is shown in Fig. 44.

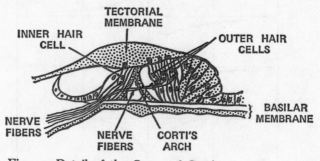

Fig. 44. Detail of the Organ of Corti.

The sensory receptors in the Organ of Corti are *hair cells.* One end of each of these cells rests on the basilar membrane. Very fine hairs, located at the other end of each hair cell, make contact with the *tectorial membrane.* A pair of rods, joined in a "V-shape," form *Corti's Arch,* which gives structural strength to the Organ of Corti. The *inner hair cells* lie on one side of Corti's Arch, the side closest to the central core around which the cochlea spirals. The *outer hair cells* are located on the other side of the arch. There are four rows of hair cells—one row of inner and three rows of outer hair cells—along most of the basilar membrane's length, from the oval window to the helicotrema. All told, there are about 3500 inner cells and 20,000 outer cells.

Signals in the nervous system, as we shall see in more detail in Chapter 6, are transmitted as electrochemical pulses along *nerve fibers*. Nerve fibers from the *auditory nerve* extend into the Organ of Corti. The endings of these fibers are very close to the sensory hair cells. When the basilar membrane vibrates in response to incoming sound waves, the hair cells are bent. In a way not completely understood, the hair cells in turn stimulate the fibers of the auditory nerve, producing electrochemical pulses that are sent to the brain along the auditory nerve.

THE PERCEPTION OF SOUND

We have examined the anatomical and physiological characteristics of the hearing organ. It is now time to consider the question, "*What* do we hear when we listen?"

This question involves the nature of our sensations when we listen to auditory stimuli. Its study is largely the province of the experimental psychologist, and forms part of the fields of psychophysics and psychoacoustics.

It is important to realize that, on the "what we hear" level, we are dealing with experiences that are purely subjective. Obtaining experimental data involves exposing a human subject to an auditory stimulus, through earphones or a loudspeaker, for example, and asking him to tell us something about the sensations it produces. For instance, we can expose him to an audible sound, gradually decrease its intensity and ask him when the sound is no longer audible. Or we can expose him to a very loud sound to determine when a sensation of pain first occurs.

Or again, we may send a complex sound through the headphone to one ear and ask the subject to adjust the frequency of a tone going to the other ear until its pitch is the same as that of the complex sound. These are a few of the many kinds of experiments that interest psychoacousticians.

Data obtained in this way is often variable. Different people, for example, have large differences in auditory sensitivity. Even the same person will respond differently on different occasions. This can depend on whether he had time for breakfast, whether he had a good night's sleep, or whether his mind is on next Sunday's football game instead of today's acoustic "beeps and boops." In addition to this inherent variability, there also are right ways and wrong ways to conduct experiments. Just as in calling heads or tails to the flip of a coin we sometimes unconsciously alternate our calls, subjects in psychoacoustic experiments tend to give patterned responses when they are unsure of what their responses should be. This all leads to a much greater degree of variability than when purely physical measurements are made.

This discussion is meant to point out some of the difficulties involved in getting reliable results from subjective experiments. Psychoacoustic experimentation is, however, the only quantitative means we have of learning how the over-all hearing mechanism responds to sound. All of the phenomena and measurements we will discuss in the remainder of this section were obtained by careful psychoacoustic experimentation.

HEARING ACUITY

Sound waves reaching the ear are simply mechanical vibrations of air particles. But all motions of air molecules are not perceived as sound. An ultrasonic "dog" whistle cannot be heard by man. A breeze that makes leaves rustle becomes inaudible as we walk away from the tree, although we still feel it. We know, almost intuitively, that sounds—to be perceptible—must be within a certain range of frequencies and intensities.

The intensity at which a sound is just distinguishable from silence is called the *absolute threshold* of hearing. In making threshold observations, experimenters work chiefly with pure tones. In one such study, conducted by the U. S. Public Health Service, a survey was made of the hearing acuity of a typical group of Americans. The results are shown in Fig. 45. The horizontal axis shows the frequency of a stimulus tone in cycles per second. The vertical axis is labeled with three different scales: first, on the right, in terms of sound pressure level (dynes per square centimeter); second, in terms of the equivalent intensity (watts per square centimeter) of the plane sound wave in free space that has the sound pressure level shown on the right; and third, in terms of decibels relative to a reference level of 10^{-16} watts per square centimeter.

Each curve in the figure is labeled according to the percentage of the group that could hear sounds weaker than the level shown by the vertical scale. For example, when a 1000 cps tone was used, 90 per cent of the group could still hear the tone when its intensity at the ear was less than 10^{-13} watts per square centimeter (or, equivalently, when its sound pressure level was less than about 0.006 dynes per square centimeter); but only one per cent of the group could hear the tone when its intensity was reduced to about 2×10^{-16} watts per square centimeter. The 50 per cent curve, indicated by a heavy line, shows that half the group could hear tones at the level indicated, while the other half needed higher intensities.

The upper curve in the figure represents the intensity

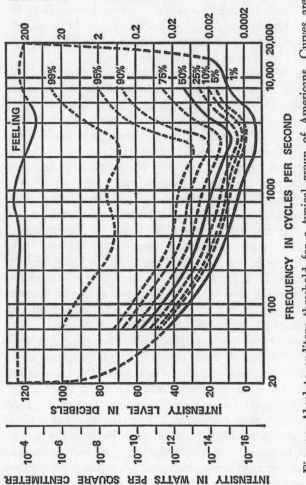

Fig. 45. Absolute auditory threshold for a typical group of Americans. Curves are labeled by per cent of group that could hear tones below the indicated level.

at which people begin to feel sound as well as hear it. When the intensity is increased beyond this level, people report discomfort and a tickling sensation. An intensity about 100 times greater than the curve of feeling normally causes definite sensations of pain, and sustained listening at these or even somewhat lower levels can do permanent damage to the ear. The useful range of hearing for any individual is usually taken to be the area between his absolute threshold and the curve of feeling. We see (in Fig. 45) that the ear's useful frequency range is between about 20 and 20,000 cps. The useful intensity range varies with frequency. For frequencies between 1000 and 6000 cps—the range to which the ear is most sensitive—tones are audible over an intensity range of some 1000 billion to one.

Because the range of intensities is so large, it is convenient to compare the relative intensities of two sounds by using the decibel scale described in Chapter 3. Table III shows the relationship between ratios of intensities and the decibel scale. We refer to sound intensities in terms of dB relative to a reference level near the absolute threshold of hearing. Although there really is no single absolute threshold, a level of 10^{-16} watts per square centimeter has been chosen for reference. Notice in Fig. 45 that on the dB scale of intensity level, the zero dB value is assigned to 10^{-16} watts per square centimeter. Other levels are marked in dB relative to this absolute threshold. For every 10 dB increase, the sound power (since intensity and power are equivalent) increases by a factor of 10.

We can now examine the enormous range of sound powers the ear is exposed to. In the following examples, it must be remembered that all intensities are relative to 10^{-16} watts per square centimeter:

At zero dB intensity, sound is barely perceptible;

An average whisper produces an intensity of 20 dB four feet from the speaker;

Forty dB is about the level of night noises in a city;

Normal conversation at a distance of three feet is usually at an intensity between 60 and 70 dB;

A pneumatic drill 10 feet away makes a 90 dB noise.

Hammering on a steel plate two feet away produces a level of 115 dB, a sound almost at the threshold of feeling. But even this amount of acoustical energy is insignificant by ordinary standards. In fact, if all the acoustic energy generated by 100 men hammering on steel plates were converted into electrical power, it would just be enough to run a 100 watt light bulb.

The eardrum, of course, is sensitive to the pressure variations in sound waves. What is the range of pressure variations to which the ear responds? The answer is indicated on the scale at the right-hand side of Fig. 45, which shows pressure levels as they correspond to the intensities shown in the left-hand scale. Thus, we can describe a sound wave in terms of pressure variations as well as energy flow.

The ear responds to remarkably minute pressure variations. The pressure level corresponding to zero dB, which is about the threshold of hearing, is 0.0002 dynes per square centimeter. Since the area of the eardrum is about one square centimeter, the total force acting on the eardrum, for sounds of this intensity, is about 0.0002 dynes. Now a dyne is a very small unit of force. To support a one-ounce weight against the force of gravity, for example, we have to exert an upward force of some 28,000 dynes. The force acting on the eardrum at the very threshold of hearing, then, is about 140 million times smaller than the force needed to lift a one ounce weight.

A force this slight hardly causes the eardrum to move from its rest position. In fact, near the threshold of hearing, the eardrum moves about 10^{-9} centimeters, or approximately one-tenth the diameter of a hydrogen molecule. Even at ordinary conversational levels, the eardrum moves only 100 hydrogen molecule diameters; and at the threshold of feeling, the motion is still only about one-thousandth of a centimeter. Motions of the basilar membrane, moreover, are about 10 times smaller than the eardrum's.

PHYSICAL VERSUS SUBJECTIVE QUALITIES

So far in our discussion, we have talked about the *intensity* (or power) and the *frequency* of a pure tone. Both are *physical* characteristics of sound and can easily be measured in the laboratory. Corresponding to these physical characteristics, but quite different in meaning, are the *subjective qualities* of *loudness* and *pitch*. The difference between the *physical* properties of a sound and the *subjective* qualities of the same sound cannot be stressed too strongly. The *physical properties* are inherent in the *sound wave* itself and can be measured independent of any human observer; the *subjective properties* are characteristic of the sensations evoked in a human listener and cannot be measured without a live listener. This fundamental distinction appears again and again in psychophysical experiments.

LOUDNESS LEVEL AND INTENSITY

Suppose we have a listener wearing a set of headphones. He has at his fingertips a two-position switch and a dial.

With the switch in the first position, he hears a 1000 cps tone at a fixed intensity, say of 40 dB. When he throws the switch to the second position, a different pure tone is fed to the earphones, say of 200 cps. By turning the dial, he can adjust the intensity of the 200 cps tone from the threshold of hearing to the threshold of feeling. He is asked to turn the dial setting until the two tones are equally *loud*. While doing so, he may flip the switch to compare the *loudness* of the two signals. Despite the fact that signals one and two sound much different, the listener usually finds it easy to choose a dial setting which, in his opinion, makes the *loudness* of signal two equal to that of signal one. However, the *intensities* of the two tones are far from identical.

Experiments of precisely this sort were used to deter-

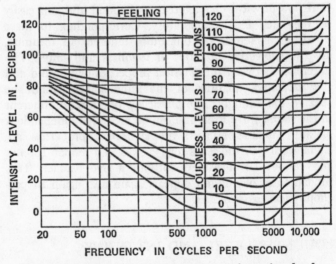

Fig. 46. Loudness level contours vs. intensity levels. Curves are labeled with loudness level measured in phons.

mine the *loudness level* contours shown in Fig. 46. The *loudness level* of a given tone is defined as the intensity (measured in decibels) of a 1000 cps tone that sounds equal in loudness to the given tone. The unit of loudness level has been named the *phon* (pronounced to rhyme with *John*). The numbers on each of the contours in Fig. 46 are the number of phons corresponding to that contour. For example, all points on the 40 phon contour are rated equal in loudness to a 1000 cps tone at an intensity of 40 dB. Thus, a 100 cps tone must be at an intensity of about 62 dB to have a loudness level of 40 phons, while a 30 cps tone of the same loudness must have an intensity of almost 80 dB.

As a second example, we notice that the contour for a loudness level of zero phons is very similar to the one per cent hearing threshold curve shown in Fig. 45. It is not surprising that all barely audible tones appear to be at the same loudness level. Finally, we see that if we decrease equally the intensity of tones of equal loudness, the resulting sounds are no longer of equal loudness.

Suppose, for instance, that we are listening to a high fidelity system at a high intensity level. If we then decrease the intensity—and, consequently, attenuate (weaken) all frequencies by an equal amount—we notice that the bass appears to be attenuated (perceptually) more than the mid- and high-frequency sounds. To be more specific, suppose both 1000 cps and 50 cps tones are sounded, each originally at a loudness of 100 phons. Assume that 30 dB of attenuation is then introduced by adjusting the volume control. We can see from Fig. 46 that the 1000 cps tone will then have a loudness of 70 phons, while the 50 cps tone will be at only 34 phons. This is the reason hi-fi fans turn up the bass as they turn down the volume. (The numerical results in our example are not exact, because Fig. 46 was measured using pure tones and does not apply directly to complex sounds; however, they are approximately correct.)

A NUMERICAL SCALE OF LOUDNESS

The *phon* scale of loudness level is an example of what psychologists call *intensive* scales. Such scales enable us to place measured sensations in rank order or, in other words, to arrange sensations in order of increasing magnitude. A tone at a level of 60 phons, for example, is always louder than a 40 phon tone, and both are louder than a 10 phon tone. But an intensive scale does not tell us *how many times* greater one quantity is than another; it tells us only that it is greater.

In addition to intensive subjective scales, psychologists have also devised subjective scales that express numerical relations between things measured. These are called *numerical* scales. In the case of loudness, the numerical scale that has been developed uses the *sone* as its unit of loudness. Listeners judge a sound having a loudness of two sones to be *twice* as loud as a one sone sound which, in turn, is twice as loud as a one-half sone sound. Arbitrarily, a loudness of one sone has been assigned to a 1000 cps tone at an intensity level of 40 dB.

Although several methods have been used to evaluate the loudness relationship, a common technique is to expose a listener alternately to two tones and ask him to adjust the intensity of one of them until it is twice as loud (or half as loud) as the other. It may seem surprising that listeners are able to do this with consistent results but, surprising or not, they can. Fig. 47 shows how the sensation of loudness (in *sones*) relates to the loudness level of a tone (in *phons*). Notice that perceived loudness is far from proportional to loudness level. For example, to

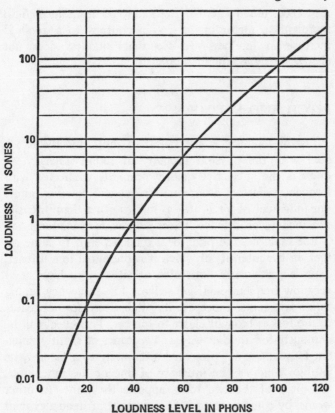

Fig. 47. The loudness function, showing how perceived loudness (in sones) depends on the loudness level of the stimulus (in phons).

increase the loudness of a sound from 0.1 sone to 10 sones (an increase of 100 in perceived loudness), we must increase the loudness level from 20 to about 66 phons. By referring back to Fig. 46, we can convert from phons directly to intensity level in dB. For example, for this 100-fold difference in perceived loudness, we must increase a 1000 cps tone by 46 dB (from 20 to 66 dB). Since 46 dB represents a factor of 40,000—in contrast to a 100-fold increase in loudness—we see that loudness does not change nearly so rapidly as intensity.

PITCH AND FREQUENCY

Just as loudness is the sensation most directly associated with the physical property of sound intensity, so *pitch* is the subjective quality primarily connected with frequency. Factors other than frequency, however, affect our judgment of pitch, just as factors other than intensity (frequency, for instance) affect judgments of loudness.

For example, the pitch of a tone depends to some extent on the intensity at which it is presented to a listener. This is particularly noticeable at either very high or at very low frequencies. If we strike a low frequency tuning fork (say, about 150 cps), its pitch decreases noticeably as the fork is brought closer to the ear. This effect can be demonstrated another way. If two tones of slightly different frequencies are presented alternately to a listener, he is able to adjust the intensity of one of the tones until the pitch of the two tones appears the same. In other words, by compensating for a difference in frequency with a difference in intensity, he makes the two tones sound of equal pitch.

For sounds with complex waveforms—as opposed to the simple sinusoidal shapes of pure tones—pitch alters only slightly as intensity changes. This is fortunate for musicians. Think how much more involved piano playing would be if one had to strike the note "D" when playing a very loud passage, but the note "C" when playing the same passage at a lower intensity!

A NUMERICAL PITCH SCALE

Frequency provides a rank order scale (an *intensive* scale, as described on p. 108) for pure tones of fixed intensities. Under these conditions, the higher the frequency, the higher the perceived pitch. A *numerical* pitch scale has been devised using techniques similar to those used to develop a numerical loudness scale. Listeners were presented alternately with two tones at a fixed loudness level; in the case to be reported here, a loudness level of 40 phons was used. One tone was fixed in frequency, while the other's frequency could be varied. The listeners were asked to adjust the frequency of the variable tone until its pitch appeared to be half that of the fixed tone. Ten different frequencies were used as the fixed tone. Remarkably enough, judging "half the pitch" is easier than one might suppose. The five subjects used in the pitch experiment showed a high level of consistency in their decisions.

The unit of pitch has been named the *mel*. On a pitch scale constructed from experiments like the one above, 1000 mels is taken as the pitch of a 1000 cps tone, 500 mels as the pitch of the tone that sounds half as high, 2000 mels as the pitch of the tone that sounds twice as high, and so on. The pitch function obtained by this process is illustrated in Fig. 48. The curve shows that our perceptual evaluation of pitch is far from proportional to the frequency of the tone producing it. For example, the tone rated at one-half the pitch of a 1000 cps tone has a frequency of about 400 (not 500) cps.

On the other hand, a tone with a pitch of 2000 mels sounds twice as high-pitched as a 1000 mel tone, but is

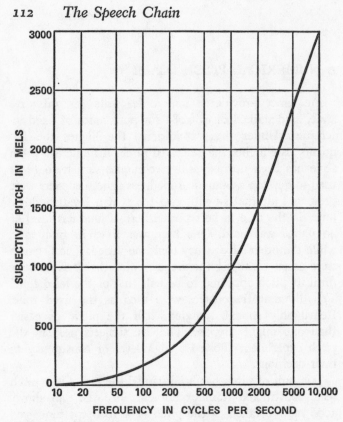

Fig. 48. The mel scale of pitch, showing how subjective pitch (in mels) is related to frequency (in cps) for pure tones.

four times as high in frequency. These results are still another example of the careful distinction we must make between the *sensations* (in this case, pitch) produced by a stimulus, and the *physical properties* (in this case, frequency) of the stimulus itself.

THE PITCH OF COMPLEX SOUNDS

Although we have defined a pitch scale in terms of pure tones, it is obvious that more complex sounds—such as musical notes from a clarinet, spoken words, or the roar of a jet engine—also produce a more or less definite pitch.

In Chapter 3, we saw that we can consider complex waveforms to be made up of many components, each of which is a pure tone. This collection of components is called a *spectrum*. For many periodic sounds—most musical and speech sounds, for example—the pitch depends on the frequency of the spectrum's lowest component. On the other hand, if observers are asked to judge the pitch of a collection of tones lying within a small frequency range, they tend to select a pitch close to the center of the band.

When a complex tone consists of several frequencies differing by a constant amount, the perceived pitch is often that of a tone whose frequency is equal to the common difference. Thus, when components of 700, 800, 900 and 1000 cps are sounded together, the pitch is judged to be that of a 100 cps tone. Or, when the component frequencies are 400, 600, 800 and 1000 cps, the pitch is judged to be that of a 200 cps tone. When tones of 500, 700 and 900 cps are added to this last collection of components, the perceived pitch drops an octave to 100 cps.

Do not be alarmed if this last paragraph has confused rather than clarified your understanding of the pitch of complex sounds. The seemingly simple problem of explaining how a sensation of pitch is produced in the hearing mechanism remains baffling to this day. Research into this problem is still going on. Some theories that explain parts of the available data will be described in Chapter 6.

DIFFERENTIAL THRESHOLDS

Earlier, we discussed the *absolute threshold* of hearing for pure tones. We defined this as the minimum intensity at which a listener could distinguish tones from silence.

We are now going to examine another threshold, the *differential threshold*, which tells us how small a change in stimulus a listener can detect. The differential threshold is frequently called a *difference limen* (*DL* for short) or *just noticeable difference* (*JND* for short). Again for convenience, we will limit our discussion to pure tones and consider the minimum detectable changes in intensity—when frequency is held constant—and the minimum detectable changes in frequency, when intensity is held constant.

Like most of the subjective characteristics of sound we have talked about, the difference limen is not a constant. It depends upon both the frequency and intensity of the tone for which it is measured. For example, a 1000 cps tone at a 5 dB intensity level—5 dB above 10^{-16} watts per square centimeter—must be about doubled in intensity, a 100 per cent increase, before a change is noticeable. On the other hand, a mere 6 per cent change in intensity is detectable in a 1000 cps tone at a 100 dB intensity level.

Suppose, instead of using ratios in the above examples, we had reckoned intensity directly in terms of watts per square centimeter. We would then say that the difference limen or differential threshold at 1000 cps is about 0.3 millionths of a billionth of a watt at an intensity level of 5 dB, and about 60 billionths of a watt at 100 dB. The 2 DL's differ by a factor of 200 million, while the corresponding fractional changes, 100 per cent and 6 per cent, differ by a factor of 33. Obviously, the differential threshold for intensity is more a fixed fraction of the stimulus than a fixed difference in intensity.

Careful measurements also have been made of the minimum detectable frequency change for tones of many intensities and frequencies. For moderate level sounds, a two to three cps frequency change is detectable in tones below 1000 cps. For tones of higher frequencies, the DL is roughly a constant fraction of the frequency, amounting to about one-twentieth of a semitone. (Two consecutive notes on a piano, black keys included, differ by one semitone; this is about a six per cent change in frequency.)

Based on measured difference limens, it is possible to compute the number of pure tones a normal listener can distinguish. For example, if the loudness level is kept at 40 phons, so that tones differ only in frequency, it appears that there are some 1400 distinguishable frequencies. This is the same as saying that the ear perceives about 1400 different pitches for pure tones at a constant loudness level. On the other hand, if the frequency is kept constant, say at 1000 cps, so that tones differ only in intensity, there are about 280 perceptually different intensity levels; that is, the ear perceives about 280 different loudnesses. If we continue computing, we can show that the total number of distinguishable tones—if both frequency and intensity changes are allowed—is between 300,000 and 400,000. If we add to this the number of different complex tones, which are undoubtedly more numerous than pure tones, we see that the ear has amazing powers of discrimination.

We must remember, however, that these figures apply only to sound comparisons made under ideal listening conditions, where two sounds are compared at a time, and pairs of sounds are presented in rapid succession.

MASKING EFFECTS

We all know that it is harder to hear sounds in noisy surroundings than in a quiet room; we shout to make ourselves heard at a football game but, in a library, the gentlest whisper can draw reproachful stares. Psychophysicists have learned a great deal about how the ear analyzes sounds by examining the way certain sounds drown out or *mask* other sounds. Although the amount of data obtained through masking experiments is enormous, we will only consider two experiments of particular significance.

First, let us see how masking experiments are conducted. The degree to which one part of a sound is masked by the rest of the sound is usually determined by making two threshold measurements. The part of the sound that does the masking is called the *masker* component; the part masked is simply the *masked* component. We begin by finding the intensity at which the masked component is just audible above the masker; this is its *masked threshold*. Next, we find the intensity at which the masked component is just audible when sounded alone; this is its *absolute threshold*. The ratio of these two intensities, expressed in decibels and called the *threshold shift*, is taken as a measure of masking.

Extensive studies have been made of the masking effects of pure tones. It was found, of course, that these effects vary greatly with frequency and intensity. But two extremely interesting results stand out. First, for moderate masker intensities, tones tend to mask most effectively other tones of neighboring frequencies, rather than tones far removed in frequency. Second, low frequency tones effectively mask high frequency tones, but high frequency tones are much less effective in masking low frequency tones.

Experiments have also been conducted in which noise was used to mask pure tones. As we learned in Chapter 3, we can consider noise to be the sum of many sinusoidal components. Consequently, when a pure tone is sounded against a background of noise, it is very much as if it were being masked by many pure tones simultaneously. As we might expect, the most effective maskers are the noise components closest in frequency to the masked tones.

The importance of these results will become apparent in Chapter 6, where we discuss theories of how the hearing mechanism operates.

BINAURAL EFFECTS

All the experiments we have talked about were performed either by applying a sound stimulus to one ear or by applying identical sounds to both ears. In normal hearing situations, sound waves that reach one ear differ from those received by the other ear. They differ primarily in two respects. First, there is a difference between signal intensities at the two ears; second, there is a difference between the times at which each ear receives corresponding portions of the sound waves.

Perhaps the most important binaural effect is the localization of sound sources. (*Binaural* simply indicates the use of both ears.) Under normal circumstances, we have no trouble telling the direction a sound comes from. For example, we can locate a source of low frequency tones to within about 10 degrees.

In localizing sound, we use the aforementioned differences in arrival times of sound waves and their differences in intensity. We can demonstrate this by a simple experiment in which sound from the same source is fed independently to each ear through earphones. Electrical networks are used to make the sound reach the right ear a few milliseconds (thousandths of a second) before or after it arrives at the left ear. The sound reaching the right ear can also be made more or less intense than the sound at the left ear.

When the sounds are equally intense and arrive at each ear simultaneously, the apparent location of the sound source is directly in the center of the head. However, if we delay the sound going to the right ear, the sound source seems to move toward the left ear. If we now increase the intensity of the sound in the right ear, the sound source will again appear to be centered in the head, and not on the listener's left side. We see that in sound localization, a difference in arrival time at the two ears can be compensated for by appropriate differences in intensities.

Binaural hearing also helps us to separate interesting sounds from a background of irrelevant noise. In a room where several conversations are taking place, for example, it is easy to "tune in" on one of them and ignore the rest. Undoubtedly, our binaural sense of direction plays a part in this.

Finally, it might be mentioned that stereophonic recording systems represent an attempt to restore the listener's sense of "presence," his sense of actually being at a performance. This is largely lost in monophonic recordings. One such stereo system uses two microphones placed several feet apart; sound vibrations reaching each microphone are recorded separately. The recording is played back over two speakers spaced several feet apart. Sounds recorded by each of the microphones are played back separately through the speakers. When we listen to a stereophonic recording, the sound does not appear to come directly from either of the speakers, but seems to be spread over a wide area. Individual instruments seem to be located at particular places, just as they would be in a concert hall, and we find it easy to concentrate on certain instruments and ignore others. In contrast, when we listen to monophonic (single loudspeaker) recordings, it is as if we were listening through a "hole in a wall" between ourselves and the performers, with all the sound coming from one point.

One drawback of stereophonic reproduction is that, to hear its full effect, listeners must be equally distant from each of the loudspeakers, essentially on an axis halfway between the speakers and perpendicular to the line joining them. "Off axis" listening tends to emphasize the sounds coming from one of the speakers, although the stereophonic effect can still be appreciable.

Chapter 6

NERVES, BRAIN AND
THE SPEECH CHAIN

Consider the roomful of electronic equipment that makes up a modern, high-speed digital computer. Rack after rack of transistors, diodes, magnetic core memories, magnetic thin film memories—all laced together by an intricate system of wiring many miles in length. Imagine the room, and everything in it, shrunk to about the size of a cigarette package. Now suppose we give this marvelous box to a clever electrical engineer—a man working, however, not in our own midcentury, but about the year 1900. We present our gift and demonstrate a few of the remarkable feats it can perform: several hundred thousand additions in one second, the translation of a Russian sentence into English and the singing of a song, complete with a piano-like musical accompaniment. We leave this tantalizing device with the suggestion that he try to find out what's inside the cigarette package; how the essential components work, how they are interconnected and organized and how they function as a complete system.

The prospects for our friend are less than bright. But it is this sort of problem that faces scientists in search of knowledge about the structure and functioning of the human nervous system and the brain. Some progress has been made, a remarkable amount considering the difficulty of the task. A great deal is known about the anatomy of the nervous system. The basic building block of the nervous system, the neuron, has been identified and studied in great detail. But the complete story of how any single function of the nervous system is carried out still remains a mystery. Exactly what takes place in your brain as you read this sentence? How do you associate each written word with an idea learned long ago? What complex mechanism causes your eyes to follow the written line across this page? We can formulate an endless stream of questions to which satisfactory answers are unknown.

Questions about the part the nervous system plays in the processes of speech, hearing and conscious thought are relevant to our subject of spoken communication. Thought is organized at the highest levels of the nervous system. Concepts are put into words, and commands are sent that cause appropriate movements of the muscles controlling the speech organs. On the hearing side, acoustic waves are coded—in the cochlea—into a form usable by the nervous system. After processing in the nervous system, the listener perceives these coded signals as words that convey the speaker's meaning.

In order to understand how the nervous system can carry out this complex task, it is necessary to know something about its anatomy and physiology. We will begin by considering the nature of the nerve cell or *neuron*. Billions of neurons are interconnected to form an integrated nervous system that can perform the various functions necessary for maintaining life and for carrying out man's intellectual activities.

After describing the neuron's anatomy and chemistry, we turn to a discussion of the nature of the electrical signals they carry. Next, we cover briefly the peripheral and central nervous systems, and then return to a more direct consideration of the nervous mechanisms chiefly involved in speech and hearing. The chapter concludes with a section devoted to theories of hearing. These theories attempt to relate what we hear (psychoacoustic data) to the anatomy and physiology of the peripheral hearing organs and the nervous system.

NEURONS—THE BASIC BUILDING BLOCKS

A living cell is a small, usually microscopic, mass of protoplasm enclosed in a semipermeable membrane. Materials essential for maintaining the cell's life can enter through this membrane, and waste products can pass out. Living organisms vary in complexity from simple, single-celled creatures to animals made up of billions of cells. In complex organisms, different groups of cells perform different functions and, in the course of evolution, these groups have taken on different forms that enable them to perform their specific tasks more efficiently. Man's nervous system consists of a large number (about 10 billion) of specialized cells, called neurons, woven together into a highly complex network.

Neurons appear in various forms, but certain features are common to all of them. Fig. 49 shows a more or less typical neuron. The structure shown is similar to certain neurons whose cell bodies are located in the spinal column and whose fibers extend to muscles throughout the body.

The neuron has an expanded part, the *cell body*, which contains the cell *nucleus*. Extending from the cell body

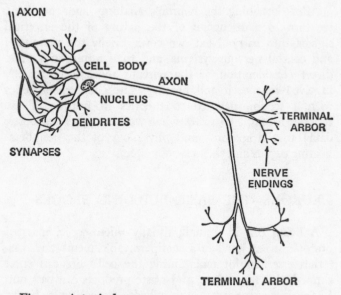

Fig. 49. A typical neuron.

is a fine filament, the *axon* or *nerve fiber*. The axon may run for a long distance, sending off several *sidebranches* along the way, before it terminates in an even finer network of filaments, the *terminal arbor*. Man's longest axon runs for several feet, from the spinal column to muscles that control movements of the toes. In spite of its great length, this axon, like all nerve fibers, is part of a single cell. It is living matter. Sever the fiber, and the portion disconnected from the life-sustaining cell body will shrivel and die.

Connections between neurons are made primarily at junctions called *synapses*. Synapses appear in diverse forms. A common type occurs where the nerve endings from the terminal arbor of one axon come into close contact with fine *dendrites*, extensions that sprout from the cell body of a different neuron. In another type of synapse, nerve endings appear to make contact directly with the cell body of a second neuron. Regardless of the precise structure, it is through such synaptic junctions that activity in one nerve cell initiates activity in a succeeding neuron.

In addition to the nervous system's neuron-to-neuron junctions, synapses also occur between neurons and *receptor cells* and between neurons and *effector cells*. Receptor cells, such as the hair cells in the Organ of Corti, receive sensory information from their environment and help to code this information into the electrochemical pulses that are transmitted and processed in the nervous

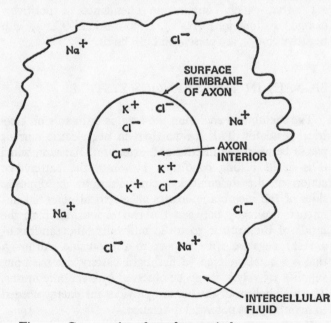

Fig. 50. Cross-section through a typical axon.

system. Effector cells, such as those in muscle fibers, respond to the electrochemical pulses sent to them along nerve fibers. In the case of muscles, the response is a contraction of the fiber.

One final aspect of the neuron's anatomy—an essential one for an explanation of its electrical properties—is the fine *surface membrane* in which it is enclosed. This membrane effectively maintains a difference in chemical constitution between the neuron's interior and exterior.

A cross-section through a typical axon is shown in Fig. 50. The interior of the axon is a jelly-like substance containing a significant concentration of positively charged potassium ions (symbolized K^+). The axon passes through intercellular fluid, very similar in composition to sea water, which contains an abundance of positively charged sodium ions (Na^+). Chlorine ions (Cl^-), with negative charge, are present in both fluids.

SIGNALS IN THE NERVOUS SYSTEM

The membrane enclosing the axon is ordinarily an electrical insulator. This means that no net electric current passes between the interior and exterior of the axon when it is in its resting condition. However, the battery-like action of the different ion concentrations on opposite sides of the membrane creates an electrical potential difference (voltage) between the two regions. In fact, the inside of the axon is 50 to 80 millivolts (thousandths of a volt) negative with respect to the outside. Although this is a small voltage (a flashlight battery, for example, supplies 1.5 volts), it can be observed by electronic means. The metabolism of the neuron provides the energy needed to maintain this potential difference.

If a neuron remained in its inactive condition indefinitely, it would be of little use to the nervous system. When it is stimulated strongly enough, however, its delicate ionic balance is upset. A rapid exchange of ions takes place between the inside and outside of the surface membrane. This motion of charged particles constitutes an electric current. The action is self sustaining, and a pulse of electrical activity propagates along the axon. It should be emphasized that energy is not transmitted from one point to another over the axon, but rather a point of local electrical activity moves along the fiber. The principal flow of current during nerve pulse conduction is at right angles to the direction of pulse propagation.

It is possible to observe the electrical character of the pulse directly by inserting a micro-electrode (a very fine electrode) into the axon, and recording the potential difference between the interior of the axon and the surrounding intercellular fluid. Fig. 51 shows the form of the observed voltage, called the *action potential*. Prior to the arrival of the action potential pulse, the axon is at its resting potential of about −60 millivolts (with respect to the potential of the intercellular fluid). When the pulse arrives at the electrode's position, the potential changes,

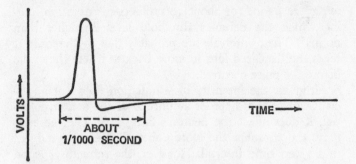

Fig. 51. The form of the nerve impulse or action potential.

and the axon becomes about 40 millivolts positive. After the pulse passes, the potential gradually returns to its resting level. Axonal conduction never takes place without this electrical activity. In general, the mechanisms involved in producing the resting and action potentials are only partially understood.

Certain properties of nerves and nerve impulses impose limitations on the way information can be coded in the nervous system. First of all, a nerve fiber is essentially an "on-off" device. If a neuron is stimulated very gently, no impulse is sent along the fiber. In order to obtain a response, the stimulus must be increased to the neuron's *threshold* level. Above this level of excitation, the neuron will fire and send a pulse along its axon. Once the threshold level has been exceeded, the shape and amplitude of the pulse is relatively independent of the intensity of the stimulation. In this sense, a nerve pulse carries no information about the intensity of the stimulus, other than that it was larger than a certain threshold value.

After a neuron has fired, there is an *absolute refractory period*, about one or two milliseconds long, during which a new pulse cannot be produced, regardless of how intense the stimulation. Following this, there is a *relative refractory period*, of about 10 milliseconds duration, during which the neuron's threshold level is higher than normal. These intervals are probably due to the time it takes the displaced ions to move back to where they were before the pulse occurred.

Although the intensity of stimulation does not appreciably affect the shape or amplitude of the action potential, it does affect the neuron's firing rate. The more intense the stimulus, the more pulses the neuron produces in a given time interval. However, the refractory period imposes a limit on the number of pulses that can be produced each second. Once the nerve fiber reaches its maximum rate, further increases in stimulus intensity have no effect. Some fibers can be fired at rates as high as 1000 pulses per second, while others have maximum rates considerably less than this. Since the pulses move along the axon with a finite velocity, several pulses may travel along a fiber at the same time.

The velocity at which a pulse travels along a nerve fiber of the type shown in Fig. 49 depends upon the diameter of the axon; the larger it is, the faster the propagation. Some nerve fibers in man are less than two microns in diameter (a micron is a unit of length equal to one-thousandth of a millimeter; for comparison, the wavelengths of visible light lie between about 0.3 and 0.7 microns). Along these fine fibers, pulses travel only a few feet per second. Neurons as large as 0.1 inch in diameter exist in some lower animals like the squid. Here, nerve pulses move about 40 feet per second.

The large nerve fibers in man (and other animals) are coated with a layer of a fatty substance, the *myelin sheath,* which is an electrical insulator (see Fig. 52). In many of man's fibers, this sheath is interrupted periodically by *nodes of Ranvier,* where very short lengths of the axon membrane are exposed. The speed of propagation along such noded fibers is much higher than the speed along

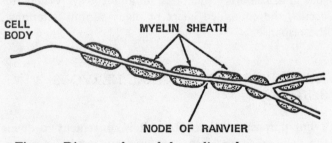

CELL BODY

MYELIN SHEATH

NODE OF RANVIER

Fig. 52. Diagram of a noded, myelinated axon.

other axons. The nerve impulse travels along these fibers by jumping from one node to the next, but the process is not completely understood. Apparently, an ionic current flow—similar to that described earlier—takes place at each node. Velocities over 300 feet per second have been observed in these axons. Noded fibers represent a great advance in the nervous system's wiring. They do not appear in lower forms of life and seem to be a comparatively recent evolutionary development.

Dendrites and nerve endings (see Fig. 49) are not sheathed in myelin. Through these fine branches, activity is transferred from one nerve to the next, but the process is not completely understood. It is clear that transmission across most synapses is accomplished by chemical, rather than electrical means. When a pulse arrives at a nerve ending, a small amount of "transmitter substance" is released, and the chemical action of this substance on the succeeding neuron tends to fire it or prevent it from firing.

Synaptic junctions, therefore, may be either *excitatory* or *inhibitory*. At an excitatory junction, a pulse arriving through a nerve ending tends to make the succeeding neuron fire. At an inhibitory junction, an arriving pulse tends to prevent the succeeding neuron from firing. A given neuron may be stimulated through several inhibitory and excitatory junctions simultaneously. When this occurs, the combined effect of many stimuli determines the response.

PERIPHERAL AND CENTRAL NERVOUS SYSTEMS

For purposes of description, it is convenient to divide the nervous system into *peripheral* and *central* portions.

The central nervous system consists of the brain and spinal cord. The peripheral system consists largely of bundles of nerve fibers that link all portions of the body to the central nervous system. These bundles, containing thousands of individual axons, are commonly called *nerves*. The fibers running in the peripheral nerves can be classified—according to function—as either *sensory* or *motor*.

The sensory fibers are concerned with the transmission of impulses initiated by an external stimulus. The first elements directly affected by such a stimulus are called receptors; for example, light stimulation causes sensory receptors in the retina to initiate nervous conduction. Impulses are then carried toward the central system along the sensory fibers of the optic nerve. Or, an acoustic stimulus reaching the ear is transformed, in the sensory receptors of the cochlea, into auditory nerve impulses that are sent to the brain.

The motor fibers of peripheral nerves are responsible for getting nerve pulses to areas of the body where they can cause muscular movements. Other fibers of the peripheral system run to organs of the body, such as glands, where they can control the activity of these organs.

The *central nervous system*, consisting of the *brain* and *spinal cord*, is the mass of nerve cells and nerve fibers responsible for coordinating and directing a great deal of human activity. Messages from peripheral receptors are brought to the central system by sensory nerves. The central nervous system sorts out and interprets these messages and initiates appropriate action; instructions are sent along motor nerves to the body's effector cells. Of course, activity can originate in the central nervous system—in intellectual activity, for example—without the necessity of direct external stimulation.

There is much evidence that the central nervous system

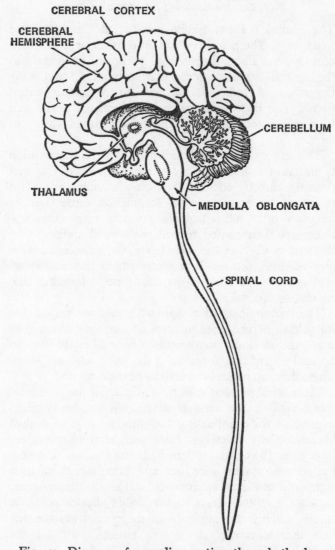

CEREBRAL CORTEX

CEREBRAL
HEMISPHERE

CEREBELLUM

THALAMUS

MEDULLA OBLONGATA

SPINAL CORD

Fig. 53. Diagram of a median section through the human brain and spinal cord.

is organized along hierarchical lines. In passing up from the spinal cord through the different levels of the brain (see Fig. 53), the structure becomes more and more complicated. Undoubtedly, this is associated with the fact that, while the spinal cord itself is concerned with relatively elementary activities, such as automatic reflex responses, the higher levels contain elaborate controlling mechanisms that coordinate the activities of the lower levels. The *medulla oblongata*, for example, at the upper end of the cord, provides reflex mechanisms for the respiratory, circulatory (heart and blood vessels) and digestive systems. The *cerebellum* receives information regarding body position and movement, and regarding muscles and their movements. It influences muscle tone and coordinates movements that may have been initiated elsewhere in the central system.

The *cerebral hemispheres*, with their many deep convolutions (folds), are probably the structures that first come to mind when one visualizes the brain. They are concerned with controlling many of the lower functions, as well as with memory, consciousness and voluntary activities. The hemispheres probably represent the peak of complexity that evolutionary development has attained. In no other organism have they acquired the size or the wealth of interconnections that they have in man.

The great concentrations of neurons in the folded surface layer of the brain are known as the *cerebral cortex*. These cells, plus the neurons in some of the lower structures, make up the brain's "gray matter." Most of the tracts of axons that interconnect various portions of the brain are covered with myelin and, because of their appearance, are called the "white matter."

FROM THOUGHT TO SPEECH

The mechanism of speech production was described in some detail in Chapter 4. It should have been apparent that speaking is a highly complex activity. Skilled movements must be made by the tongue and lips. Coordinated muscular activity takes place in areas not consciously connected with speech production, such as the chest and stomach. All of this is done so easily that we are hardly aware of the process; it seems to proceed with no conscious effort. Indeed, we are frequently involved in several other activities simultaneously—watching the scenery flash by while driving a car, for example.

But speech is much more than just a complex motor activity. It involves an acquired knowledge of the language code by which words are associated with objects and concepts. It involves a knowledge of syntax and grammar. It involves the continual interaction of stored information and voluntary conscious activity on the highest levels of the brain. In short, speech differs from most motor activities because it requires much greater efforts of the central nervous system.

The final results of the speech process, so far as the central nervous system is concerned, are streams of nerve pulses sent to control the muscles of the organs used during speech. But what patterns of nervous activity correspond to the thoughts that form in our minds prior to speaking? How do our brains store the vast amount of information necessary for speech? How do we gain access to this information when we want it—and ignore it at other times? Answers to these and many other questions are still unknown.

Neural mechanisms involved in speech production are

poorly understood largely because speech involves high
level central mechanisms; knowledge about the coordina-
tion of activity at this level of the brain is practically non-
existent. It is worthwhile at this point to consider how
scientists have learned about the structure of the brain
and nervous system, and how they are now trying to learn
the details of how they function.

Knowledge of the structure (anatomy) of the nervous
system is relatively easy to obtain. Animal and human
post-mortem dissections, carried out by many careful
workers during the past century, have provided detailed
knowledge of the gross anatomy of the nervous system;
for example, where various nerve fibers originate and end,
what types of synaptic connections exist, and what individual neurons look like.

Knowledge of nervous system functions is much more
difficult to obtain. To observe the nervous system actually
working it is necessary to use live subjects for experimentation. By using animals, such as cats and monkeys, neuro-
physiologists have made observations of the nervous activity caused by various forms of stimulation. Electrodes
have been inserted in different parts of the auditory pathway to observe nerve pulses that result from acoustic
stimulation. Electrodes that measure potentials in the
brain have been used to "map" areas of the brain that
seem to be essential for certain functions, such as hearing,
vision, or motor activity.

In animal experimentation, scientists can deliberately
remove or destroy particular areas of the brain. Or they
can sever some of the communicating cables of the nervous system. By observing changes in the animal's responses to various types of stimulation, as well as by
observing changes in its general behavior, it is possible to
learn something about the functions of various localized
areas of the nervous system.

Experiments and observations have also been made on humans. For example, observations of gross electrical activity in the brain can be made very simply by using external electrodes to record voltages at several points on the surface of the head. The result is a conventional electroencephalogram (EEG), from which scientists are able to detect and, to some extent, localize certain kinds of abnormal cerebral activity. EEG's can be taken quickly and with no danger to the patient.

Major surgery is required to observe electrical activity in localized areas inside the brain. Brain surgery always involves considerable danger to the patient and is not undertaken without very good reasons. It is performed only as a last resort on patients whose maladies are severe; for instance, when brain tumors must be removed. Or, persons suffering from epilepsy may be so incapacitated that brain surgery is worth the risk.

Disorders of the nervous system and brain because of congenital defects or disease are not so rare as we might hope. In addition, the development of human civilization has lead to many artificial ways of producing damage to the brain (and other parts of the body); for example, modern weapons, such as the rifle, the hand grenade and the automobile. Thus, there have been large numbers of cases made available—naturally and unnaturally—for study.

Once the skull has been opened surgically and the brain exposed, it is possible to observe electrical activity by inserting electrodes into the brain matter. This may be only normal background activity, or it may be activity in response to an external stimulus, such as a sound or a pin prick; or it may be produced by a conscious voluntary act on the part of the patient, such as moving a finger or speaking. The patient can be conscious during an operation of this sort because the brain itself has no receptors to report sensations of touch, heat, or pain. No more than a local anaesthetic for the scalp is necessary.

Reports on the reactions of patients to localized electrical stimulation in parts of the brain make fascinating reading. One gets the feeling of being very close to the essential nature of the human intellect, although the way it works remains a deep mystery. A patient may respond by moving an arm or finger, without knowing why he did so. He may consciously want to say something, but be completely unable to set his vocal organs into action. Or, again, he may want to name an object shown to him, but not be able to recall the object's name while his brain is being stimulated electrically. Although he is completely unaware of the electrical excitation, he recalls the word he was seeking immediately after the stimulation is stopped.

As a result of such direct experimental evidence, it seems safe to say that certain localized areas of the cerebral cortex are essential for speech production and comprehension. Removal of or damage to these areas results in a loss of the ability to communicate verbally. Usually, other aspects of the intellect are also impaired. On the other hand, large volumes of the brain sometimes can be removed without noticeably impairing speech or other functions. What this all implies in terms of brain structure and organization is not completely understood.

HEARING AND THE NERVOUS SYSTEM

While the speech process begins at a high level in the central nervous system, the hearing process (so far as the nervous system is concerned) begins in the inner ear at the hair cells. The ultimate perception of the "heard" event takes place, of course, in the brain. The signals received at the ear are transmitted over an intricate pathway of nerves to their destinations in the sensory centers of the cerebral cortex. Some information processing undoubtedly takes place at synaptic junctions along the way.

The cell bodies of the receptor neurons, about 28,000 in each ear, are located in the *spiral ganglion,* which runs parallel to the Organ of Corti. It can be seen in Fig. 54.

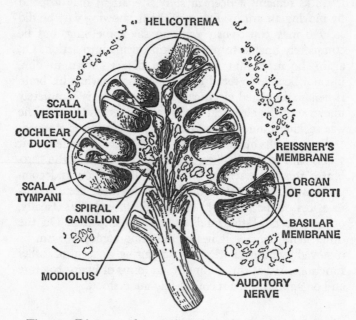

Fig. 54. Diagram of a section through the core of the cochlea.

Axons from these cell bodies pass inward to the *modiolus,* the cochlea's hollow core. Here, they form the neat bundle of fibers known as the *auditory nerve.*

Dendrite-like extensions run from the spiral ganglion's cell bodies into the Organ of Corti, where their endings make synaptic contact with the sensory hair cells. Fibers frequently make connections with many hair cells, and each hair cell typically receives extensions from more than one nerve fiber. Although most of the fibers are sensory—carrying information toward the central nervous system—there is evidence that some of them carry signals from the brain to the Organ of Corti. This arrangement constitutes a complicated feedback loop through which the brain can somehow exercise control over conditions at the peripheral hearing organs.

No nerve fiber extends all the way from the Organ of Corti to the auditory area of the cerebral cortex. Connections with other nerve fibers are made at several synapses along the way. The principal pathways to the cortex (for auditory stimuli) are shown in Fig. 55. Axons originating in the spiral ganglion make their first synaptic connections with fibers of the central system in the *cochlear nucleus*. Each fiber coming from the spiral ganglion seems to make connection here with 75 to 100 cells. Since the total number of cells in the cochlear nucleus is only about three times the number of cells in the spiral ganglion, each cochlear nucleus cell receives connections from many incoming fibers. There are many cell types and many types of axon endings to be found here. Very little is known about the information processing that takes place on this or higher levels.

From the cochlear nucleus, axons run in a nerve bundle, called the *trapezoid body*, to the next mass of cell bodies in which synaptic connections are made. This mass of cells is called the *superior olivary complex*, due to its olive-like shape. From here, fibers proceed upward through pathways that can be seen in Fig. 55. There is no need to name them all. From the figure, which is of course very schematic, it can be seen that fibers occasionally bypass some of the cell masses and arrive at a given level after passing through fewer than the normal number of

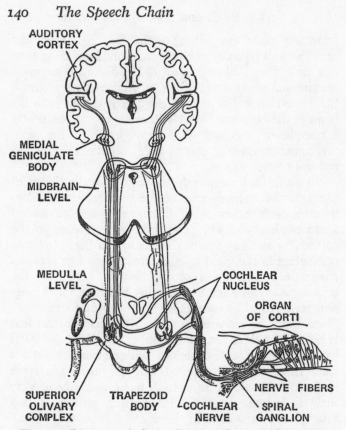

Fig. 55. Diagram of the auditory pathways linking the brain with the ear.

synapses. It should be noted that a similar descending nervous pathway exists, through which pulses originating in the brain can travel back to the ear.

At the thalamic level in the brain is the *medial geniculate body*. This mass of cells is the last stopping point before the highest level of the brain. Fibers arrive here from lower in the auditory pathway. From this point, nerve fibers proceed directly to the auditory projection area of the sensory cortex.

THEORIES OF HEARING

The sensations we experience are somehow generated by the nerve pulses that flow to and circulate in our brains. A most complicated form of information processing takes place, but we can do little more than marvel at its results. Our understanding of the mechanics of the ear and the peripheral sensory nerves is considerably better than our understanding of auditory mechanisms in the central nervous system.

An explanation of the perception of acoustic signals in terms of the anatomy and physiology of the hearing organs and nervous system is the major objective of auditory theory. In our brief account of auditory theory, we shall confine ourselves to three subjects: how the ear resolves a complex sound into its component tones; how loudness is determined; and how we can explain the masking experiments discussed in Chapter 5.

Early in the nineteenth century, the German physicist G. S. Ohm postulated what has become known as Ohm's acoustical law. (He is much better known for his electrical law.) He stated, essentially, that when we are exposed to a complex sound containing many pure tones, the hearing mechanism analyzes that sound into its frequency components. Thus, we are able to perceive each of the tones individually. We are not ordinarily aware of this when listening to sounds, but a trained listener can, to some extent, resolve individual harmonics in a complex sound.

In the latter half of the nineteenth century, the great German scientist, Hermann von Helmholtz, proposed a mechanism to account for this frequency analysis. By

Helmholtz's time, the development of microscopic techniques had allowed anatomists to construct a fairly accurate picture of the inner ear's structure. On the basis of this knowledge, Helmholtz suggested that the basilar membrane consisted of a great number of fibers tightly stretched across the cochlea, much like the strings of a piano. Each of these fibers was supposed to resonate at a particular frequency, depending on the fiber's tension and weight. When the fluid in the cochlea was set into vibration by motions of the stapes footplate, only those fibers tuned to frequencies present in the stimulus would be set into motion. Individual nerve fibers were supposed to run from each tuned element to the brain. The tones perceived would correspond to the resonant frequencies of the tuned fibers that were excited. This hypothesis was called the *resonance theory* of hearing.

To show the divergence of opinion that can exist when experimental evidence is lacking, we will also mention the *telephone theory* of pitch perception, which was put forward around the turn of the century. At that time, it was becoming widely accepted that transmission in the nervous system was electrical in nature, although details, such as its pulse-like character, were unknown. It was proposed that the ear simply converted acoustical vibrations into electrical vibrations, much as a microphone converts acoustic waves into electrical signals. Nerves were likened to telephone cables that simply conveyed electrical signals, unchanged in form, to the brain. All processing of information was thought to be carried out at the highest levels in the central nervous system.

Both of these theories are now known to be wrong. There are no transverse tuned fibers in the basilar membrane that function as Helmholtz suggested. Neurons do not transmit signals the same way a telephone line does. Furthermore, many of the perceptual effects implied by these theories simply do not agree with the psychoacoustic measurements now available.

The modern view of how the ear works still puts considerable emphasis on the inner ear's ability to analyze the frequencies of incoming sound waves. Although the mechanisms involved are quite different from those assumed by Helmholtz, the frequency of the stimulus *is* transformed into a *place* of maximum vibration along the basilar membrane. For this reason, we call this a *place theory* of hearing.

Evidence for a place theory is two-fold: first, direct experimental observations of the vibrating basilar membrane; second, theoretical models based on measurements of the basilar membrane's mechanical properties. From this evidence we know that, in response to a pure tone at the stapes footplate, the amplitude of the basilar membrane's vibration varies as one moves away from the oval window toward the helicotrema. A maximum vibration level is reached at a point that depends on the frequency of the stimulation. For high frequencies, the maximum is close to the oval window. For low frequencies, the maximum is closer to the helicotrema. For frequencies below about 100 cps, the maximum vibration is always at the apical end of the basilar membrane. The form of this response is shown in Fig. 56 (which is identical to Fig. 42).

Notice that, in general, the amplitude of vibration gradually increases all the way from the oval window to the point of maximum vibration; but beyond this point, the amplitude rapidly decreases.

The hair cells of the Organ of Corti are deformed by motions of the basilar membrane. Somehow, these hair cell deformations produce pulses in the nerve fibers to which they are connected.

Now consider some observations of nervous activity

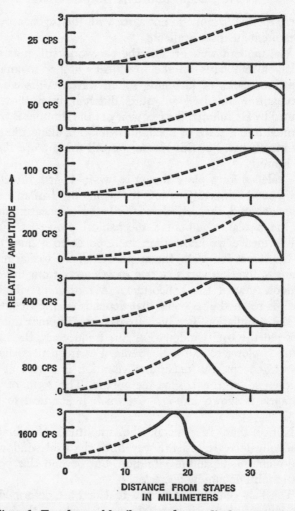

Fig. 56. Envelope of basilar membrane displacement for different frequencies of sinusoidal excitation applied at the stapes.

made with pure tone stimulation. If an electrode is placed in a single fiber of the auditory nerve, that fiber is found to be most sensitive to a tone of a particular frequency. If we assume that the individual nerve fiber receives its excitation from a particular small length of the Organ of Corti—as the anatomical evidence strongly suggests—this result is not surprising. Indeed, any individual fiber must respond most easily to the frequency that provides the strongest response at the place in Corti's Organ to which the fiber is connected. For tones of other frequencies, the intensity must be greater before the nerve cell fires.

Frequency selectivity is not very great in fibers of the auditory nerve. Typically, a fiber is readily excited by tones lower than its characteristic frequency, provided that the stimulation is moderately above threshold. But for tones somewhat higher than its characteristic frequency, it is difficult to get the fiber to fire. The reason for this can be inferred from Fig. 56. Suppose we are looking at a nerve fiber that is most sensitive to 400 cps tones. According to the figure, its endings must terminate about 24 millimeters from the stapes. The 24 mm point responds to some extent to all tones lower than 400 cps. However, for a 1600 cps tone, the 24 mm point hardly moves for the level of stimulation shown, and it would take a tremendous increase in stimulation to get it to move appreciably. For frequencies of excitation higher than those shown in the figure, the basilar membrane response becomes even more localized and closer to the oval window.

The character of responses in fibers higher in the auditory pathway—for example, in the medial geniculate body —is considerably different. Many cells can be found that do not respond to pure tone stimulation, regardless of frequency, but do respond to clicks or noise. This is unlike the behavior of auditory nerve fibers, which will respond to a pure tone stimulus, provided its frequency is correct and its intensity is above threshold. Other neurons have been found—in both the medial geniculate body and in the auditory portion of the cortex—that do respond to pure tones. They seem to be much more selective than auditory nerve fibers and the cells of the cochlear nucleus. They respond to only a narrow band of frequencies centered about their characteristic frequency.

The present view, then, is that the perception of tone pitch depends to some extent on *which* fibers carry pulses to the brain; but there is undoubtedly more to the process than this simple place mechanism.

It is believed that loudness, on the other hand, is related to the total number of pulses reaching the brain's auditory areas each second. The more intense the sound stimulus, the larger the number of pulses triggered in the inner ear and transmitted to the brain. Specific details of the process are not known. The fact that different fibers have different thresholds may play an important role. Feedback paths from the brain to the ear may cause thresholds to vary, depending on conditions existing at a given time, and complicate matters even more.

Finally, we should comment on the pure tone masking effects described in Chapter 5. You will recall that pure tone masking refers to the ability of one tone to drown out or mask a second tone. We emphasized two major effects: first, that a tone most effectively masks other tones of neighboring frequencies, rather than tones far removed in frequency; second, that low frequency tones effectively mask high frequency tones, but high frequency tones are much less effective in masking low frequency tones. Both these effects are explainable, qualitatively, in terms of the place mechanism behavior of the basilar membrane.

We have seen that a tone causes the entire basilar membrane to vibrate, but that the amplitude of vibration is largest at a particular place along the membrane. The place of maximum vibration depends on the frequency of the tone. As we might expect, a very weak tone, just above the hearing threshold, is barely able to cause a neural response. This response is highly localized and occurs very near the basilar membrane's place of greatest motion. Vibration of the membrane elsewhere is not sufficient to fire the nerve fibers that end there.

If a masking tone considerably above threshold is presented to a listener, neural responses occur over a fairly large length of the membrane. In fact, responses will occur wherever the amplitude of vibration provides greater than threshold stimulation of the nerve endings. At points close to the place of maximum vibration, there will be considerable nervous activity. Furthermore, at points where frequencies higher than the masking tone would produce their maximum effects (that is, at points closer to the oval window), there is appreciable vibration due to the masking tone. But at points where lower frequencies would produce a maximum response (that is, at points closer to the helicotrema), there is little activity.

Now consider what happens when we add a weak tone, of different frequency, to the masking tone, and present this new stimulus to a listener. At places where the basilar membrane is not vibrating appreciably (that is, at places corresponding to frequencies lower than the masking tone), the threshold for neural stimulation should be the same as if the masking tone were not present. Thus, low frequency tones are not masked effectively by high frequency tones.

At points where the basilar membrane is vibrating strongly (that is, at places corresponding to frequencies near and above the masking tone), the presence of the additional component of the stimulus will not be detected until it is strong enough to change the pattern of vibration significantly. We see, then, that neighboring or lower frequency tones do mask high frequency tones. In a qualitative sense, the place theory is in good agreement with observed masking effects.

Chapter 7

THE ACOUSTIC
CHARACTERISTICS OF SPEECH

Our vocal organs produce a wide variety of sound waves. The way they produce such waves was described in Chapter 4. The way the sound waves affect the human hearing mechanism was explained in Chapters 5 and 6. In this chapter, we will consider measured characteristics of these waves.

Much of the available data concerns their intensity levels and their spectra. The waveshapes, an obvious target for study, are not often investigated. Indeed, listening experiments have shown that speech recognition is often unaffected by large changes in waveshape.

THE INTENSITY LEVEL OF SPEECH

The acoustic energy of normal speech is surprisingly small. Our vocal cords can convert only a fraction of the energy of the air stream flowing from our lungs into acoustic energy—about one-twentieth of one per cent, in fact. The energy of a speech wave during one second of speech is only about 200 ergs; it takes a billion ergs to keep a 100 watt bulb lighted for the same one second span.

When we speak, the available sound energy is scattered in all directions. In normal conversational speech—some three feet from the speaker—the average sound intensity is half-way along the scale of audible sounds. It is about a million times stronger than the weakest audible sound and about one million times weaker than the strongest sound we can hear without feeling discomfort. This intensity is 65 dB greater than 10^{-16} watts per square centimeter, the intensity of a just audible sound. It corresponds to a pressure variation of about one-millionth of normal atmospheric pressure. The varying sound pressures of speech, then, are only a very small fraction of the air pressure that always surrounds us.

The pressure and intensity values just mentioned were obtained by averaging several seconds of speech. Characteristically, the intensity of speech varies considerably about this average value. Even if we ask someone to speak steadily at a normal conversational level, the speech intensities produced vary greatly as he pronounces speech sound after speech sound. There is roughly a 700-to-1 range of intensities between the weakest and strongest speech sounds made while speaking at a normal conversational level. The vowels are the strongest sounds but, even among these, there is a three-to-one range. The strongest vowel is the "aw" (as in "*ta*lk"), which is usually pronounced at three times the intensity of the weakest vowel, "ee" (as in "*see*"). The strongest of the consonants, the "r" sound, has about the same intensity as the "ee" vowel, but is two and a half times more intense than "sh" (as in "*sh*out"); six times more intense than "n" (as in "*n*o"); and 200 times greater than the weakest consonant, "θ" (as in "*thin*"). This considerable range of intensities is produced when a person speaks at what he and his listeners consider to be a constant level. Of course, greater intensity variations will be observed as we go from speaker to speaker. A survey of the telephone conversations of a large number of persons showed that the *average* conversational speech intensity they produced varied over a range of about 100-to-1; from 75 dB to 55 dB, relative to the reference intensity of 10^{-16} watts per square centimeter.

There also are intensity variations as we move from loud shouting, through normal conversation, to quiet speech. The range is from 85 dB through 65 dB to 45 dB. When we whisper, our average speech intensity may drop another 10 or 20 dB.

Measuring the intensity of connected speech has brought to light another feature of our speaking habits. We rarely speak without making frequent pauses, sometimes for only a fraction of a second, at other times for several seconds. Quite often, we make "ah" and "uh" sounds, which are really pauses in the continuity of producing meaningful speech. Psychologists are investigating these pauses, and are finding interesting relations between the pattern of pauses and the speaker's personality.

THE SPECTRUM OF SPEECH

The speech spectrum is concerned with the frequency and intensity of each overtone (harmonic) of the speech wave. Even 19th century speech scientists were aware of the important contributions these overtones make to intelligibility. Over the years, therefore, many investigations of the speech spectrum have been made.

We are obviously interested in the spectrum of each

individual speech sound, and we will have much to say about this later in the chapter. First, however, let us see what is known about the over-all spectrum produced when the effects of all speech sounds are combined. In this kind of analysis, we use a long sequence of connected speech—a sequence long enough for every sound to occur many times. The energy level in each part of the spectrum is measured and summed up separately for the whole speech sequence. The summated energy for each part of the spectrum is then plotted. The resulting curve is the *long time average speech spectrum* in Fig. 57. It shows

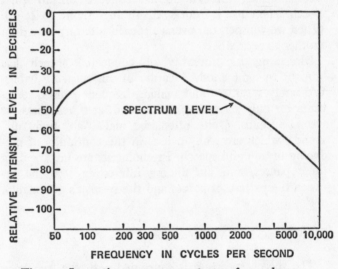

Fig. 57. Long time average spectrum of speech.

that speech energy is generated roughly from 50 to 10,000 cps. The energy is greatest in the 100 to 600 cps region, which includes both the fundamental component of the speech wave and the first formant. Above these frequencies, the energy decreases until, at 10,000 cps, it is

50 dB below the peak level that occurs around 300 cps.

A considerable amount of spectral information is also available about individual speech sounds, particularly for the vowels.

The most significant features of the vowel spectrum are the frequencies and amplitudes of the various formants. These, you will recall, correspond to the resonances of the vocal tract, and they produce peaks in the speech spectrum. Even though a certain amount of ingenuity is sometimes required to identify the spectral peaks caused by vocal tract resonances, the spectrum is our best guide for finding these important formants.

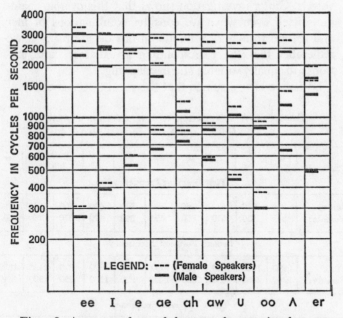

Fig. 58. Average values of formant frequencies for 10 English pure vowels. The vowels were spoken in isolated single syllable words.

Usually, the first three or four formant frequencies are adequate for recognition. These are given in Fig. 58 for 10 English pure vowels. The values shown are the average frequencies obtained from the speech of a number of male and female speakers. The vowels were pronounced in one syllable words, like "heed" and "hid," and each syllable was spoken in isolation. (Table VI is a tabulation of the values displayed graphically in Fig. 58.) The variability of the formant frequencies is shown in Fig. 59, where individual results are plotted, rather than averages. We see that the range of formant frequencies produced when any one vowel is uttered overlaps the ranges of adjacent vowels. Closer investigation shows that this overlap maintains itself even when we consider combinations of first and second formants. This should not be surprising if we remember that the corresponding articulatory configurations are equally variable and overlapping.

So far we have assumed that the vocal tract—and, there-

TABLE VI—A TABULATION OF THE AVERAGE FORMANT
FREQUENCY VALUES SHOWN IN FIG. 58

	ee	ɪ	e	ae	ah	aw	ʊ	oo	ʌ	er
First Formant Frequency										
Male:	270	390	530	660	730	570	440	300	640	490
Female:	310	430	610	860	850	590	470	370	760	500
Second Formant Frequency										
Male:	2290	1990	1840	1720	1090	840	1020	870	1190	1350
Female:	2790	2480	2330	2050	1220	920	1160	950	1400	1640
Third Formant Frequency										
Male:	3010	2550	2480	2410	2440	2410	2240	2240	2390	1690
Female:	3310	3070	2990	2850	2810	2710	2610	2670	2780	1960

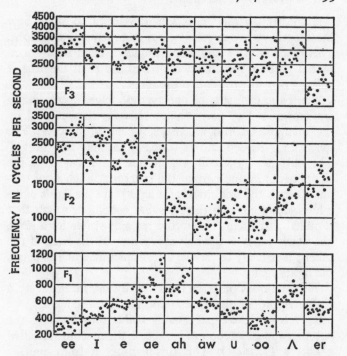

Fig. 59. The formant frequencies of 10 English pure vowels as pronounced by a number of different speakers. (The notations, F_1, F_2 and F_3 refer to the first three formant frequencies.)

fore, the speech spectrum—remains in a certain fixed shape while one speech sound is being produced, and changes rapidly to the fixed shape appropriate for the next speech sound. Like the early speech scientists, we were thinking of speech as a sequence of different stationary configurations. We will see from what follows in this chapter that the speech wave has very few segments whose principal features remain even approximately static; *speech is a continuously varying process.*

A special machine has been developed to show how the speech wave spectrum varies from instant to instant. This machine, the *sound spectrograph,* plays such an essential part in speech research that we shall describe it before discussing the data it produces.

The basic elements of one type of sound spectrograph are shown in Fig. 60. The speech wave is converted by the microphone into an analogous electrical wave. The spectrum is divided into 12 bands by 12 "analyzing filters." The output of each filter indicates the strength of the components in one part of the spectrum. Each filter output controls the brightness of a light bulb; the lights make a luminous record on the phosphor coating of a belt that is pulled past them. The record remains visible for a time, but slowly fades as the belt moves around the back of the rollers; it is ready to receive a fresh picture when it passes the lights again.

The luminous patterns produced by the machine are a visible record of the speech spectrum; consequently, we often refer to these patterns as *visible speech.* Since the patterns appear as soon as we speak, the machine is called a *Direct Translator.* This distinguishes it from another version of the spectrograph, which needs a delay of five minutes to produce a visible record of the spectrum.

The latter machine divides the speech spectrum (from 100 to 8000 cps) into about 500 bands, and produces a permanent record on special paper. The construction of this type of spectrograph is different from that of the Direct Translator but, the spectral records—the *spectrograms*—produced by the two machines are similar in appearance.

Examples of such spectrograms are shown in Figs. 61, 62, and 63. In all these patterns, time is shown along the horizontal axis and frequency along the vertical. The darkness of the trace indicates the energy level of the spectral

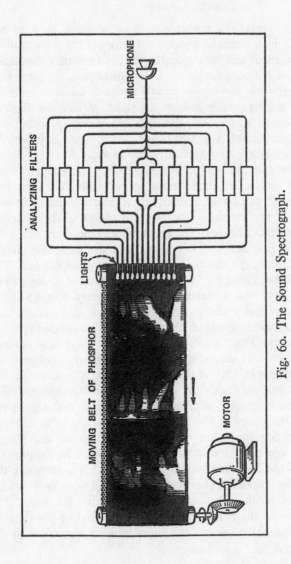

Fig. 60. The Sound Spectrograph.

components. For example, a spectral peak, such as one made by a formant, produces a dark area at a point along the vertical axis corresponding to the formant's frequency. If that formant frequency is left unaltered, we get a horizontal dark bar whose length depends on how long the formant frequency is kept constant. When the formant frequency is increased, the dark bar bends upwards; when it is decreased, the bar bends down. The dark bar disappears when we stop making the sound.

The spectrograms in Fig. 61 show what happens when pure vowels are pronounced in isolation. The first four formants can be seen clearly; they remain constant in each of the spectrograms because the vowel quality remains unaltered. The patterns for a variety of diphthongs are in the line below. They show how the formants change as the sound quality is altered during a diphthong. The third line shows how a consonant at the beginning or end of a pure vowel makes the formants vary. Fig. 62 shows how markedly the patterns vary for a spoken sentence.

The spectrogram of a sentence said at normal speed is shown in Fig. 63. We can see that the frequency and amplitude of the many spectral peaks vary continuously. For example, look at the last word of the sentence in Fig. 63: "rich" or "rɪtsh" as it would be written phonetically. At the beginning of the word, three formants are visible. The frequency of the first formant remains relatively constant, but the other two rise rapidly. Soon, the fourth, fifth and sixth formants also are visible. The frequencies of all the formants remain comparatively stable during the middle section of the word. This is followed by a sudden silence as the air flow is interrupted for the sound "t," shown by the blank segment near the end of the spectrogram. Finally, there is the fuzzy looking section when the fricative "sh" is spoken.

Looking at the whole spectrogram, the impression of

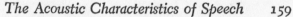

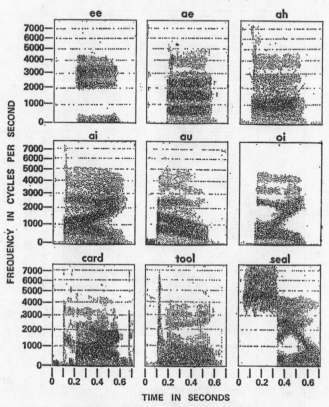

Fig. 61. Typical speech spectrograms. The sounds represented are shown above the spectrograms.

many components moving in many different ways is unmistakable. Various segments stand out from the rest and catch our eye. There are the segments with the clearly defined dark formant bars, and the very obvious closely spaced vertical lines. These vertical lines are produced only when the vocal cords vibrate. There are also the blank segments indicating the absence of any sound when the

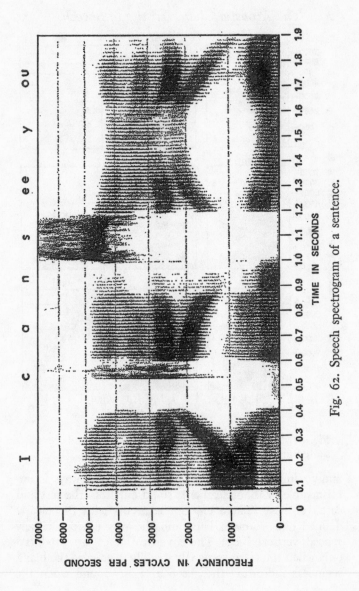

Fig. 62. Speech spectrogram of a sentence.

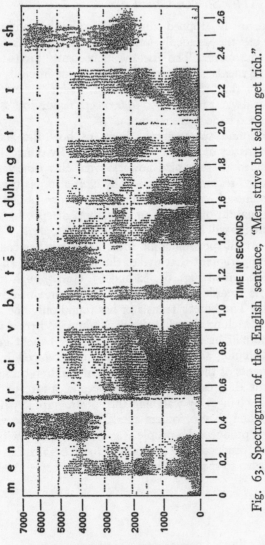

Fig. 63. Spectrogram of the English sentence, "Men strive but seldom get rich."

air stream is stopped during the plosive consonants. There are the decidedly lower intensity segments of the nasal consonants. The fricative consonants produce the fuzzy segments. They are of much lower intensity (less dark) for the "f" and "th" sounds than for "s" and "sh"; they are darkest in the 4000 to 6000 cps region for "s," and in the 2000 to 3000 cps region for "sh."

The sound spectrograph shows us how the acoustic characteristics of speech vary with time. By doing this, it has helped us recognize how essential this time-varying, "dynamic" feature of speech really is. It also has triggered a long line of experiments that have thrown much light on the nature of the dynamic features of speech. These experiments will be described in the next chapter.

Almost all spectrographic speech research has centered on the instrument that makes the more detailed spectrograms shown in Figs. 61, 62 and 63, even though it produces its records only after a delay of approximately five minutes. The Direct Translator has found only one application: teaching speech to deaf children. When children with normal hearing learn to speak, they benefit greatly from listening to the acoustic effects produced by the movements of their vocal organs. Deaf children cannot do this, but they can be helped to become aware of these acoustic changes by watching the spectrographic patterns made when they or others speak. Comparing the visible patterns produced by people who hear normally with the patterns produced by their own vocal organs can help them learn to speak intelligibly.

Chapter 8

SPEECH RECOGNITION

During speech, our vocal organs produce sound waves with many different characteristics: different intensities, different durations and different spectral components. Just because our vocal organs produce a variety of features does not mean that they are all needed for intelligibility. What conditions are necessary for satisfactory speech recognition? Are all the components of the speech spectrum essential to recognition and, if not, which are the important ones? How far can we reduce the intensity of the speech wave without undermining intelligibility? These and similar questions will be discussed in this chapter.

Experiments for pin-pointing the speech wave features important to speech recognition fall into two classes. First, there are experiments in which we use the speech waves produced by a person speaking normally. We eliminate or alter some of the acoustic features of this *naturally produced* speech, and ask someone to listen to the modified sound to determine how far its intelligibility differs from that of the original speech. In the second class of experiments, we generate a speech-like wave artificially. With little trouble, we can separately adjust each acoustic feature of this *artificially produced* speech. Consequently, artificial (*synthesized*) speech is particularly suitable for speech recognition studies. For example, we can simulate only certain of the known components of natural speech and measure their effectiveness in making sounds intelligible. This allows us to determine which of the many speech wave characteristics actually help speech recognition; help us, for example, to distinguish a "p" from a "t" or an "ee" from an "ah."

Many of the experiments we will talk about depend on our having a technique for measuring the intelligibility of speech; we will begin, then, by explaining the kind of yardstick we use to measure intelligibility, before we describe experiments with artificial and natural speech and what they tell us about speech recognition.

THE MEASUREMENT OF SPEECH INTELLIGIBILITY

How do we get a yardstick of speech intelligibility, and who is to say that one speech wave is more intelligible than another?

In a typical speech recognition test, a set of words is spoken and a listener, or group of listeners, is asked to write down, repeat or otherwise respond to the test items. We count the words correctly recognized and this number, expressed as a percentage of the total number of words spoken, is taken as a measure of intelligibility.

Tests of this kind are called *articulation tests,* and the percentage of test items correctly recognized is called the *articulation score.* The name is very misleading because an articulation test is a test of speech recognition, *not* of articulation. However, since the name is widely used, we simply must be careful not to associate it with speech articulation.

The result of an articulation test depends greatly on the circumstances under which it is carried out and on the test items used. These spoken test items can be words, sentences or individual speech sounds pronounced in meaningless syllables. A test list usually consists of no less than 20 to 25 test items that include several examples of the 38 or so sounds of English.

In an articulation test, we often use lists compiled by experts who have spent a good deal of time and effort perfecting them. Usually, a number of such lists are prepared—lists carefully selected to be of equal difficulty—so that the same list need not be used twice when the same listeners are tested repeatedly. The best known test lists are the ones prepared by the Psychoacoustics Laboratory of Harvard University. The Laboratory published a set of sentence lists and two different kinds of word lists. One type of word list is made up of *spondee* words. These are two-syllable words, like "armchair," "shotgun" and "railroad," in which each word is pronounced with equal stress on both syllables. The other type of word list consists of single-syllable words. They are selected so that the speech sounds in the lists occur with the same relative frequency as they do in spoken English. These are the so-called *phonetically balanced* or PB lists.

In everyday life, we listen to sentences or sets of sentences. Sentences, therefore, seem to be the most appropriate items for articulation tests. Nevertheless, words and meaningless syllables are frequently used in testing because of their convenience. When we use word lists, however, we must know how to relate word articulation scores to the common situations in which speech is normally used. The word articulation scores will be lower than the sentence scores because a sentence, after all, can be fully understood, even if every word in it is not correctly recognized. The relationship between word and sentence scores depends on many circumstances; as a general rule, though, normal conversation can be carried on—without too much difficulty—under circumstances where a 50 per cent word articulation score was achieved with PB or similar word lists.

Articulation tests are widely used for assessing the quality of telephones or other speech processing devices. When interpreting the significance of an articulation score, we must remember that the score tells us about only one aspect of the information transmitted by speech sound waves. It tells us how well the different words of speech can be distinguished. When listening to speech, however, we also learn about the identity of the speaker: whether it is Uncle Henry speaking or the telephone operator, whether the speaker is angry or pleased, whether he is asking a question or making a statement, and so on. The articulation score does not indicate how well the listener perceives these features. Some special telephone systems transmit speech with high intelligibility, but do not cope with these other features of the speech wave. It is often very important that we know who is speaking to us and what his attitude is; consequently, such special speech transmission systems cannot be extensively used, even though the "recognizability" of the words they transmit is very high.

Let us go on to those experiments whose purpose is to pinpoint the individual acoustic features that contribute most to the recognition of particular speech sounds.

TESTS WITH ARTIFICIALLY PRODUCED SPEECH

The Recognition of Vowels First, consider the vowels. According to long accepted doctrine, vowel sounds are *produced* by modifying the vocal cord buzz with the vocal tract resonances (formants). These resonant frequencies change as we articulate different speech sounds. It is not surprising, then, that we believe vowels are *recognized* on the basis of the formants, the frequencies of their corresponding spectral peaks. This view was suggested by vowel spectrograms, like those in Fig. 61. On these spectrograms, the most eye-catching features are the dark bars produced by the formants. There is little doubt that the formant frequencies play an important part in vowel recognition.

The spectrograms of Fig. 61 also show, however, that the vowel spectra have at least four or five obvious spectral peaks. Are they all needed for satisfactory vowel recognition and, if not, which peaks are important? We can conveniently answer these questions by generating sounds with only a few spectral peaks to see if listeners can identify the modified sounds as one vowel or the other. Electronic circuits are used to produce speech-like sounds with one, two or any number of spectral peaks; the frequencies of these resonances can be set to any value within the range of audible frequencies. Such artificial speech generators are called *speech synthesizers*.

Experiments with synthesized speech sounds have shown that the first, second and third formants are more than sufficient to identify the 11 pure vowels of English. Marginal recognition is possible with just the first two formants.

We have seen that the frequencies of the first two or three formants strongly influence vowel recognition. This does not mean that a particular combination of formant frequencies will always be recognized as one and the same vowel. A vowel can be recognized even though its formant frequencies vary over a wide range. But the same combination of formant frequencies can sometimes lead to the recognition of different speech sounds, because the range of frequencies appropriate for any one vowel considerably overlaps the range suitable for the recognition of several other vowels. This has not only been observed in experiments where a listener was asked to *identify* sounds with known formant frequencies; it also agrees well with the appreciable scatter and overlap observed in the formant frequency values produced when a speaker *pronounces* a vowel (see Fig. 59).

The formant frequencies, then, do not positively identify a vowel. Later in this chapter, we will see that no acoustic feature can completely identify a speech sound. Speech recognition is based on the acoustic features of the speech wave, but it is also powerfully affected by our expectations and by our knowledge of the speaker, the rules of grammar and the subject matter being discussed. We will take up these important aspects of speech recognition at the end of this chapter. Here, we are concerned only with the *acoustic* features that influence recognition.

We have seen that the acoustic features most important for vowel recognition are the first three formant frequencies. Because vowels can be recognized in the absence of higher formants does not mean that the higher formants have no part in recognition. In fact, there is evidence that some vowels can still be recognized when the first two formants are absent and only the higher formants serve as recognition cues. It is not unusual for the speech wave to contain several simultaneous cues to the identity of a speech sound, even though each cue on its own would be adequate for recognition. We will hear more later about these *multiple cues*.

The Pattern-Playback Much of our knowledge about the acoustic features important for consonant recognition has been obtained with synthesized speech produced by one particular machine. This is the so-called Pattern-Playback, built by the Haskins Laboratories of New York. The Pattern-Playback works like a speech spectrograph in reverse. The speech spectrograph (see Fig. 60) was described in the last chapter. When a speech wave is applied to it, it produces patterns called spectrograms, like the patterns in Figs. 61, 62 and 63, which represent the spectrum of the speech input. The Pattern-Playback, on the other hand, accepts a spectrogram-like pattern, scans it with a light beam and produces the corresponding sound wave. In normal use, the spectral patterns played back on this machine are not spectrograms of natural

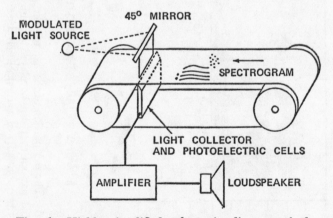

Fig. 64. Highly simplified schematic diagram of the Pattern-Playback.

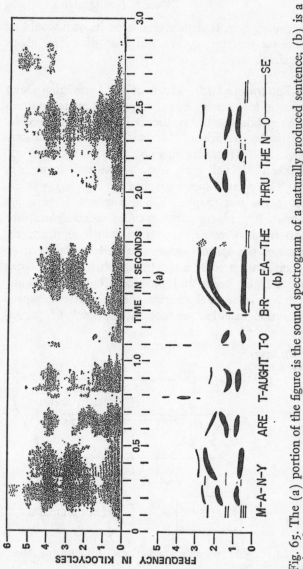
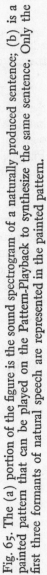

Fig. 65. The (a) portion of the figure is the sound spectrogram of a naturally produced sentence; (b) is a painted pattern that can be played on the Pattern-Playback to synthesize the same sentence. Only the first three formants of natural speech are represented in the painted pattern.

speech. Instead, we generate artificial speech by playing back similar patterns painted by hand on a plastic belt. A schematic diagram of the Pattern-Playback is shown in Fig. 64.

This artificial speech has a distinct, synthetic quality, but can still be recognized as speech. The "natural" quality of synthesized speech depends somewhat on the amount of spectral detail we paint on the plastic belt. Usually, only the first three formants are painted to get intelligible, but rather unnatural sounding speech. Fig. 65(a) is the spectrogram of a naturally pronounced sentence; (b) is the painted pattern that can be played on the Pattern-Playback to hear the same sentence.

Patterns can be painted to generate a great variety of sounds. The number of formants, their frequencies, and their durations, can be altered at will, and the different features of the sound wave changed—one at a time—to observe their effect on speech recognition.

The first experiments with the Pattern-Playback concerned the vowels and their formants. Spectral patterns were painted to include several formants, which were kept constant throughout the duration of the test sounds. When played on the machine, the patterns were heard as steady vowels, like "eee" or "aaah." As you might expect, it was found that the presence of just the first three formants was sufficient to identify the 11 pure vowels of English.

The Recognition of Plosive Consonants In painting patterns for the Pattern-Playback, it was found that a very short vertical mark, like any of the three shown in Fig. 66, was heard as a "plop"-like sound. Because of its similarity to the sound we hear when a plosive consonant (a "p," "t" or "k") is pronounced, this "plop"-like sound is often called a *plosive burst*. The perceived character of the

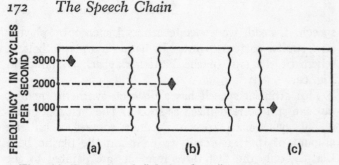

Fig. 66. Example of "plosive burst" patterns for the Pattern-Playback.

plosive burst made by the Pattern-Playback depends on the frequency at which the burst is centered. In Fig. 66 (a), the burst is centered at 3000 cps; in (b), at 2000 cps; and in (c), at 1000 cps.

Test syllables were generated from patterns in which a plosive burst was combined with a vowel section made up of two formants, as shown in Fig. 67. Many test patterns were made combining each of the 11 different vowel formant configurations with plosive bursts centered at a number of different frequencies. The test syllables generated by the Pattern-Playback were presented to a group of listeners. They were asked whether they heard the syllables as "tah," "pah" or "kah," as "too," "poo" or "koo," and so on. On the whole, no single plosive burst was consistently heard as the same plosive consonant. For example, a plosive burst centered at one frequency was heard as a "k" when associated with one vowel, and as a "p" when associated with another vowel. In other words, the kind of plosive consonant we hear depends not only on the frequency of the plosive burst, but also on the nature of the following vowel. This finding is of great importance; we will discuss it further as soon as we have described another related experiment.

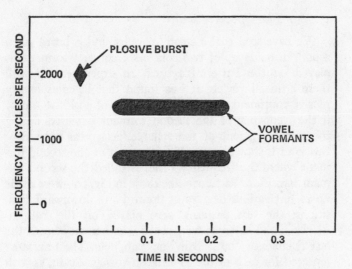

Fig. 67. A painted pattern which, when played on the Pattern-Playback, is heard as a plosive consonant followed by a vowel.

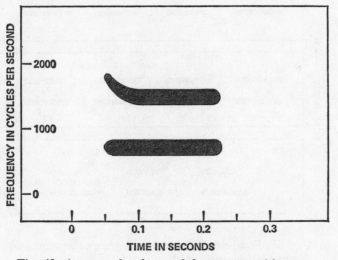

Fig. 68. An example of second formant transition.

We have seen that a steady vowel sound is heard when a pattern made up of two constant frequency formants is played on the Pattern-Playback. In experimenting with these artificial vowels, it was found that listeners hear a plosive consonant (even in the absence of a plosive burst) if the frequency of the second formant is varied during the initial segment of the syllable. A typical pattern of this kind is shown in Fig. 68. The part of the second formant where the frequency varies is called the second formant *transition*. Patterns—like those in Fig. 69—were made up to test various degrees of upward and downward transitions; the test patterns were played on the Pattern-Playback and listeners were asked whether they heard the test syllables as "tah," "kah" or "pah," etc. The tests were repeated for each of the 11 English vowels. Again, as with

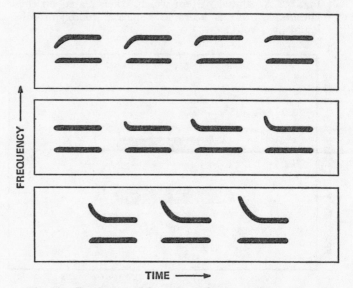

Fig. 69. Formants with various degrees of upward and downward transition.

the plosive bursts, it was found that the same kind of transition was heard as one plosive consonant or another depending on the vowel that followed.

More precisely, it was found that all the second formant transitions perceived as one particular plosive pointed toward (but never reached) one and the same frequency. This is shown by the composite sketch in Fig. 70, where we see all the second formants which, when heard on their own (combined with the first formant in

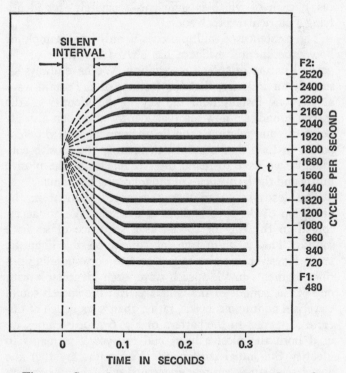

Fig. 70. Second formant transitions perceived as the same plosive consonant, "t."

the lowest part of the figure), were perceived as the consonant "t" followed by a vowel.

For the other plosives, the second formant transitions pointed toward different frequencies; about 700 cps for "p," and, usually, about 3000 cps for "k."

These results give one more example of a general property of speech, a property we have already mentioned in connection with vowel recognition, namely, that the speech wave can contain several simultaneous cues (the plosive burst and the second formant transitions, in this case), each of which is sufficient—separately—for identifying a particular speech sound.

The existence of multiple cues is only one example of how experimental evidence has altered our views of the general nature of speech recognition. We have always assumed, for instance, that the features of the sound wave at any one instant hold the key to the identity of the speech sound; we now see that identification can also depend on our relating acoustic features at two different points in time. For example, to identify the plosive consonants, we have to relate the frequencies of the plosive bursts and the frequencies of the following formants.

This leads us to another unexpected element in the operation of the speech chain as a whole. We are accustomed to thinking of speech as a sequence of separate sounds. This is quite true, of course, on the linguistic level. However, we also expect to find corresponding distinct segments in the speech wave, each identifiable with one of the sounds of the language. But the speech sound wave is a continuous event, rather than a sequence of discrete segments. In the pattern of Fig. 67, for example, we used both the plosive burst and the vowel formants to identify the initial consonant. We cannot say that the vowel segment is entirely concerned with the recognition of either the initial consonant or the following vowel.

Somehow or other, in the transition from the linguistic to the acoustic level, the sequence of *discrete* speech sounds is transformed into a *continuous* speech sound wave; we can no longer always identify one segment of the speech wave with just one linguistic unit, or vice versa.

We have now described how second formant transitions and plosive bursts serve as cues for identifying plosive consonants. How about the acoustic cues for recognizing the fricative sounds?

The Recognition of Fricative Consonants Unquestionably, we distinguish fricatives from all other sounds by the "hissy" noise the turbulent air stream produces. This turbulence shows up on speech spectrograms as a fuzzy segment. Many experiments have shown that air turbulence, whether produced by the vocal organs or simulated by a speech synthesizer, is heard as a fricative sound. But what are the cues for distinguishing one fricative consonant from another; for example, for distinguishing "s" from "sh" and "sh" from "f"? Experiments with both natural and synthetic speech indicate that we distinguish the "s" and "sh" sounds from other fricatives because the intensities of these two are greater than those of the rest. We distinguish "s" from "sh" by spectral differences; we hear "s" when most of the fricative energy is concentrated in the spectral region above 4000 cps, and we hear "sh" when the energy is concentrated in the 2000 to 3000 cps region.

The weaker fricatives, the "f" and the "θ," are distinguished more by the nature of their neighboring vowels' second formant transitions than by the spectral shape of the fricative segments themselves. In other words, we hear a "θ" sound when the neighboring vowel's second formant transition is appropriate for a "θ"; the spectrum of the fricative segment is less important, so long as its intensity is low.

The duration of the fricative segment also matters; if it is shortened considerably, it sounds like a plosive consonant. We can tape record a normally pronounced word ("see," for example) and cut short the duration of the initial fricative segment (by literally cutting out the corresponding length of tape). If we reduce the length of the fricative segment to about one-hundredth of a second (from its original length of approximately one-tenth of a second), we hear the word "tee."

Formant Transitions and Place-of-Articulation We have already mentioned the importance of second formant transitions as cues for distinguishing plosives and for distinguishing the fricatives, "θ" and "f." They play an equally important part in distinguishing nasal consonants. Fig. 71 shows the patterns which, when played over the Pattern-Playback, are heard as "pah," "tah," "kah," and "mah," "nah," and "ngah." We can see that the second

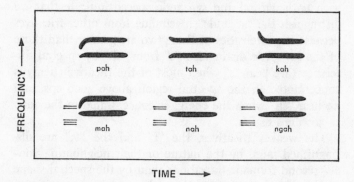

Fig. 71. Patterns showing the relationship between second formant transition and place-of-articulation of consonants.

formant transitions are identical for "pah" and "mah," for "tah" and "nah" and for "kah" and "ngah." The pairs of syllables differ only by what precedes the vowel segments: silence in the case of the plosives, and a low intensity buzz (heard vaguely as nasality) for the nasals. The syllable pairs with *identical second formant transitions* are heard as consonants with the *same place-of-articulation*. We conclude, then, that one way we can identify a consonant's place-of-articulation is by the nature of the second formant transition of its adjoining vowel.

The Effect of Duration We have already seen that the duration of the fricative segment of a speech wave can distinguish plosives from fricatives—a "t" from an "s," for example. Further experiments with the Pattern-Playback have provided additional examples of the important part duration can play in speech recognition.

Several examples of a two-syllable word—like "object" —were synthesized; the patterns of formant frequency variations for all test words were identical. This means that the first syllables of all test words had identical formant frequencies. Similarly, the formant frequencies of all the second syllables were the same. The durations of the syllables, however, were different in each of the test words. In some words, the vowel in the first syllable was made longer in duration than the second vowel; in others, the second vowel was made longer than the first vowel. The words with the longer first vowel were heard with the stress on the first syllable, as in "(the) *object*." When the second vowel was longer, listeners heard the stress on the second syllable, as in "(to) *object*." The experiment shows that the duration, rather than the intensity, of the vowel segments can determine which syllable is heard stressed.

The shift of stress from one syllable to the other had another effect. Listen to someone say the words, "(the) *object*" and "(to) ob*ject*." You will find that the vowel in the first syllable is pronounced differently in the two words. The same feature appeared in experiments with synthetic words. When the first syllable was short, listeners heard the "uh"-like quality of an unstressed vowel. When the syllable was long, as in "(the) *object*," they heard the "ah" sound appropriate for the stressed syllable. In brief, listeners identified two sounds with *identical formants* as different vowels, depending on duration. The way vowel quality is influenced by duration is still another important new aspect of speech recognition brought to light by experiments with the Pattern-Playback.

Artificial speech has been used in many other experiments. We have said enough, however, to show the usefulness of the Pattern-Playback and other synthesizers in identifying the acoustic cues necessary for speech recognition.

We will now describe what we have learned about speech recognition from experiments with naturally produced speech.

TESTS WITH NATURALLY PRODUCED SPEECH

Natural speech has been used in tests to establish the general conditions required for speech recognition: the intensity ranges over which speech remains intelligible, the amount of noise that can be tolerated before recognition is affected, and so forth. In other experiments, we eliminate or distort certain acoustic features of natural speech. We then compare the intelligibility of the original and modified speech waves to assess the significance of the eliminated or distorted features for speech recognition. We will consider such experiments one by one.

The Effect of Intensity First, over what range of sound intensities is speech intelligible? To find out about this, the average intensity of a speech wave was increased in steps, starting at a level low enough to make speech inaudible. At each intensity level, a word articulation score was obtained. The results are shown on the graph of Fig. 72. We see that speech becomes fully recognizable

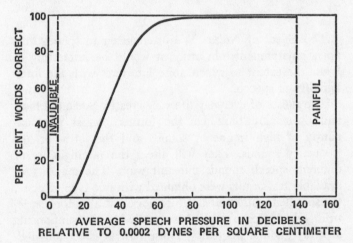

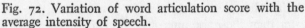

Fig. 72. Variation of word articulation score with the average intensity of speech.

(a word score of about 50 per cent) for an average intensity of 30 or 40 dB stronger than 10^{-16} watts per square centimeter (the absolute threshold of hearing). This barely intelligible speech is about equal in intensity to a whisper at three feet. Speech remains fully intelligible until its intensity becomes high enough to cause pain. Understandably enough, at such levels, listeners are more concerned with pain than with recognizing words. The graph shows that speech is intelligible over the amazingly wide intensity range of some 80 dB (100 million-to-1).

The results shown in Fig. 72 refer to average intensities. The individual speech sounds become intelligible at different *average* speech levels. Vowels are heard at lower average levels and, among the consonants, the "θ" (as in "*th*in") will be heard last. We expect this because the intensity of vowels is greater than that of consonants when we speak at a constant average speech level (see Chapter 7).

The Effect of Noise We often listen to speech in a noisy environment; obviously, it would be interesting to know the extent to which noise interferes with the intelligibility of speech.

The noises of everyday life vary greatly. Some are hissy and others are buzz-like; the former consist predominantly of high frequency sounds and the latter of low frequency sounds. They will affect the intelligibility of different speech sounds different ways. The majority of available test results were obtained with one type of noise, the so-called *white noise*. White noise has a uniform spectrum, which means that it has equally intense components at every audible frequency. Noise has no effect on intelligibility when the speech intensity is more than 100 times greater than the noise intensity. (This is called a 100-to-1 signal-to-noise ratio.) A 50 per cent word articulation score is obtained when the average intensities of speech and noise are about equal (one-to-one signal-to-noise ratio). In everyday life, however, speech is often intelligible even when its intensity is lower than that of noise. For example, if noise and speech come from different directions, our perceptual mechanism somehow manages to separate the two. This helps when we want to recognize speech in a noisy situation: a busy street, for example.

Experiments with Filtered Speech A great variety of experiments have been performed with natural speech to find *which* of the wide range of frequencies generated by the vocal organs are essential for speech recognition. In such experiments, we measure the intelligibility of speech heard over a transmission system that responds to only a limited range of frequencies. We alter the range of frequencies the system can deal with and observe the effect on speech recognition.

Devices that respond to only certain frequencies are called *filters*. We can have *low pass* filters, *high pass* filters or *band pass* filters. A low pass filter transmits all sound wave components whose frequencies are below a certain "cut-off" frequency. For example, a low pass filter with a 1000 cps cut-off frequency transmits all components of the input wave whose frequencies are less than 1000 cps, but weakens components above 1000 cps. Similarly, a high pass filter with a cut-off frequency of 800 cps transmits all components whose frequencies are higher than 800 cps, but weakens those below 800 cps. A band pass filter has an upper and lower cut-off frequency and transmits effectively only those components whose frequencies are between the two. In the experiments we are about to describe, the filters had adjustable cut-off frequencies.

Speech is highly recognizable when heard through a low pass filter with a very high cut-off frequency. After all, a high cut-off frequency means that most components of the speech wave are transmitted. More and more of the high frequency components are eliminated when we lower the cut-off frequency of the low pass filter; consequently, the articulation score decreases. This is shown by the curve marked *LP* (low pass) in Fig. 73. With a high pass filter, the articulation score is high for a low cut-off frequency and decreases as the cut-off frequency is increased. This is shown by the curve marked *HP* (high pass) in Fig. 73.

On examining the two curves of Fig. 73, we see that they cross over at around 1800 cps, where the articulation

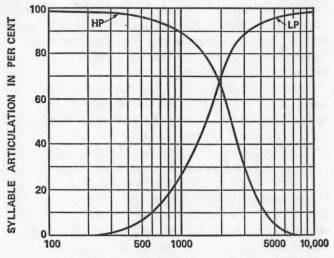

CUT—OFF FREQUENCY IN CYCLES PER SECOND

Fig. 73. Articulation scores obtained with filtered speech. (The curve marked HP refers to high pass filters; LP refers to low pass filters.)

score for both curves is 67 per cent. We must remember that this 67 per cent score was obtained with meaningless syllables, and that normal conversation is fully intelligible under such conditions. Fig. 73 indicates, then, that we can follow a conversation when we hear only those components of the speech wave below 1800 cps. But speech is equally intelligible if all these low frequency components are eliminated and we hear only the components above 1800 cps.

Further experiments show that we need neither all the low frequency nor all the high frequency speech components for satisfactory intelligibility. A band pass filter can be used to select a restricted range of speech frequencies. The band of frequencies may be taken from anywhere in the speech spectrum and, in each case, the filter's upper and lower cut-off frequencies can be adjusted until good intelligibility is achieved. Tests like this show that although this minimum bandwidth is different at different parts of the spectrum, a surprisingly narrow band of frequencies is always sufficient for satisfactory recognition. In the range around 1500 cps, for example, a 1000 cps bandwidth is sufficient to give a sentence articulation score of about 90 per cent. Other experiments show that intelligibility is even higher when we hear the speech frequencies between about 100 cps and 3000 cps.

Experiments with Distorted Speech The effect of waveshape distortion has also been investigated. The speech waveshape can be severely distorted by a process called *peak clipping*. The diagram in Fig. 74 shows that peak clipping does just what its name implies: it clips off the peaks of the speech wave. The clipping level can

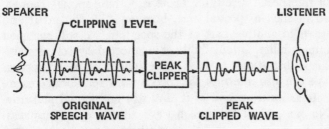

Fig. 74. An explanation of peak clipping.

be set as low as one or two per cent of the speech wave's original peak values. Under these circumstances, the intricately shaped speech wave is transformed into a sequence of square pulses. Of course, this drastic distortion considerably alters speech quality but, surprisingly enough, word articulation scores of 80 and 90 per cent can still be obtained. In other words, even severely peak-clipped speech remains highly intelligible.

Frequent interruptions also modify the speech waveshape. Let us assume that the speech wave is switched on and off at regular intervals, and that the duration of each interruption is always equal to the duration of the intervals during which speech is allowed to pass. When speech is interrupted at a slow rate—"on" for one second and "off" for the next—whole words are lost and intelligibility is poor. But when the rate of interruption is increased (to more than 10 interruptions per second), the word recognition score rises to around 90 per cent. This means that even though we can hear the speech wave for only half the time, we still find it highly intelligible. However, just as with so many of the distortions we have discussed, the quality of interrupted speech is poor.

We have seen that the speech wave is intelligible over a wide range of intensities, and that it remains intelligible in the presence of even large amounts of noise. The speech wave is intelligible even if we listen to only part of the speech spectrum. There is nothing special, though, about such a spectral area, because if we discard it and listen to another part of the spectrum, we still get good intelligibility. Intelligibility is unaffected by severe waveshape distortions, such as those caused by peak clipping. We can also interrupt the speech wave periodically, eliminate as much as half of it, and still understand perfectly. No one part of the speech wave, therefore, is indispensable for satisfactory speech recognition.

These results may be unexpected and surprising, but we will see that they fit into the over-all picture of the speech recognition process. We can now try piecing together such an over-all picture by combining all we have learned about speech and its recognition.

ESSENTIAL INGREDIENTS FOR RECOGNITION

In earlier sections of this chapter, we learned about those characteristics of the speech sound wave that serve as cues for distinguishing speech sounds. Some of these acoustic features are spectral, like the frequencies of formants, plosive bursts and fricative segments. Other features, like formant transitions, are concerned with the relationship of spectral features at different instants of time. Important cues are provided by the duration of certain segments of the speech wave, and others by speech wave intensity (for differentiating "s" and "sh" from "f" and "θ," for example).

Experiments in speech recognition *and* production have shown, however, that these cues are highly variable. A wide range of formant frequencies is recognized as the same vowel, and the ranges appropriate for each vowel overlap. We have observed the same effect in examining the formants produced when vowels are pronounced. The formants for any one speech sound vary from speaker to speaker; they are also greatly influenced by the sounds that precede and follow them. It is impossible to say, therefore, that a particular vowel is invariably associated with a particular combination of formant frequencies.

Experiments with filtered and distorted speech have shown that acoustic cues are not only ambiguous, but that we can actually eliminate many of them and still get good speech recognition.

How do we recognize speech when the cues are so highly variable or when many of the cues are eliminated? Part of the explanation is that there are *multiple* acoustic cues for recognizing many of the speech sounds. We eliminate one, but the others remain. This is far from sufficient, however, to explain the remarkable ease and certainty with which we recognize the ambiguous and often distorted acoustic cues provided by the speech wave in everyday conversation.

A better explanation of the way we recognize speech is that the speech wave's acoustic features are not the only cues available for speech recognition. We have already had one example of how the general speech situation—the context—influences recognition. When we described articulation testing, we mentioned that the sentence articulation score is usually higher than the word articulation score. When listening to sentences, we have certain expectations of what words we will hear. Since these contextual cues are not available when we listen to unrelated, isolated words, our understanding drops off.

There are other examples of how strongly our expectations influence our ability to recognize speech. For example, articulation tests were carried out *under comparable acoustic listening conditions* with test vocabularies of 2, 4, 8, 16, 32 and 256 English words. The listeners knew the test words; consequently, their expectations were much stronger when the test vocabulary consisted of only a few words. The test results in Table VII show that—under certain acoustic conditions—speech recognition can change from a state of almost total nonrecognition to one of almost complete intelligibility when the variety of test words is reduced from 256 to two.

Such results fit in well with our everyday experiences. You may have tried to follow a conversation under difficult listening conditions—a noisy party, for example. You probably noticed, under these circumstances, that your understanding was better when you were familiar with the subject matter than when you were not. In other words, the acoustic cues of the same piece of speech are clearly recognizable by a person familiar with the subject matter, but not by someone who has fewer expectations about the words spoken.

TABLE VII—THE EFFECT OF EXPECTATION ON SPEECH RECOGNITION. (The articulation scores obtained under comparable conditions with test vocabularies of different sizes.)

Number of Single Syllable Words in Test Vocabulary	Articulation Score
2	87%
4	69%
8	57%
16	51%
32	39%
256	14%

Similar effects can be observed in a subway station or an airline terminal. The high noise levels at these places make it difficult to understand public-address announcements. Although the same acoustic cues are available to all passengers—since they are all listening to the same speech waves—some understand the announcements, but others do not. People who travel frequently know the names of the stations or departure gates being announced. Consequently, they usually understand the announcements perfectly, while the occasional traveler looks around in bewilderment. These examples show that familiarity with subject matter can make speech intelligible even when the acoustic cues alone—because of noise, indistinct articulation, and so forth—are ambiguous and not sufficient for recognition.

Many other cues contribute to speech recognition. We know from experience how the articulation of a certain sound may be slurred (and the acoustic cues made ambiguous) by the articulatory positions required for neighboring sounds; and we know how much slurring to expect for various talking speeds. We may also have learned the articulatory peculiarities of the speaker and how to make allowances for them. (This is why it is often easier to understand a speaker we know well.)

Most important of all, we know the language we are listening to: we know its phonemes, its words and its grammar. We know what phoneme sequences make up meaningful words and how the rules of grammar and semantics determine word order.

Few people realize how narrowly these rules restrict the order in which phonemes can follow one another, and how strongly our knowledge of possible sequences helps us fill in any gaps in a stream of words we hear. For example, look at the simple English rhyme below, where all the vowels have been replaced with asterisks:

M*R* H*D * L*TTL* L*MB H*R FL**C* W*S
WH*T* *S SN*W

You probably had no trouble understanding the sentence, although about one-third of the letters are missing. Try this one:

TH* S*N *S N*T SH*N*NG T*D**

We can go much further and omit some of the consonants, too:

S*M* W**DS *R* EA*I*R T* U*D*R*T*N*
T*A* *T*E*S

You can experiment yourself to see how well we can guess missing letters just from our knowledge of the language and the identity of a few letters in a sentence. Select a sentence at random and ask a friend to guess its first letter. Count the number of times he makes mistakes before finding the right letter. Repeat the same test for the next letter in the sentence, and so on. The

```
611111   11   11  117111111   205541   6911z111
SPEECH   IS   AN  IMPORTANT   HUMAN    ACTIVITY
```

Fig. 75. An example of the importance of context. Numbers above the letters indicate the number of guesses a subject made before guessing the right letter.

results of a similar experiment are shown in Fig. 75, where you can see the sentence and, above each letter, numbers indicating the number of guesses made to find the right answer.

We see that three-quarters of the letters were guessed correctly on the first try, even though the person guessing had no preliminary information about the subject matter.

These examples show that we can recognize many words without any acoustic cues at all. We can recognize them because we know the language, and because we know what words are possible and what word sequences grammar and meaning allow. When we listen to speech under normal conditions, we get many acoustic cues, perhaps ambiguous, as well as the linguistic cues we noticed in the "guessing game." As a supplement to ambiguous acoustic cues, linguistic information serves as a powerful aid in speech recognition. In a way, the additional information restricts our choice of speech sounds, words and sentences, and these restrictions make the ambiguous acoustic cues less ambiguous. We may not know, for example, whether a sound heard in isolation is an "ee" or an "oo;" but if this same sound is heard in the middle of a word, preceded by an "sh" and followed by a "p," we will have no doubt that the vowel is an "ee," because the word "sheep" is possible in English, but the word "shoop" is not.

Speech recognition is accomplished by combining acoustic, linguistic, semantic (the subject matter, the meaning of the words spoken) and circumstantial (speaker identity, etc.) cues. When we listen under the most favorable conditions, the cues available are far in excess of what is actually needed for satisfactory recognition. Indeed, general context is often so compelling that we know positively what is going to be said even before we hear the words. This is why—under normal conditions —we understand speech with ease and certainty, despite the ambiguities of the acoustic cues. It is also the reason that intelligibility is maintained to such an astonishing extent, despite the variability of speakers and the presence of noise and distortion. Many people think that only acoustic cues make speech recognition possible; we now see that they are just one among many other important cues.

Chapter 9

A LOOK TOWARD THE FUTURE

Looking back over the previous chapters, it is clear that research performed during the past few decades has deepened our understanding of the processes involved in spoken communication. It is equally clear, however, that our present understanding is at best incomplete and, at worst, incorrect. Undoubtedly, some of what we now believe to be true will someday be as outdated as Helmholtz's resonance theory of hearing is today.

This is as it must be, for science is a vital, dynamic activity, not a static body of established truths. Only the rare, exceptional hypothesis remains for later generations to admire and accept as scientific fact. Most scientific work does not stand up to the test of time. T. H. Huxley, an eminent 19th century biologist, put it this way: "It is the customary fate of new truths to begin as heresies and end as superstitions." Or, to quote him again, "The great tragedy of modern science [is] the slaying of a beautiful hypothesis by an ugly fact."

Research has a dual effect on human affairs. First, it

leads to a better understanding of the world around us. Second, this better understanding usually leads to the development of practical applications that directly affect our everyday lives. The X-ray machine, the television set and the atomic reactor resulted from advances in technology that were based on advances in fundamental scientific understanding. In our present age of science and technology, the time lag between a scientific discovery and its impact on society is often very small. In the rest of this chapter, we will indulge our fancies and consider some of the applications to which further advances in our understanding of speech, hearing and the nervous system may lead.

SPEAKER IDENTIFICATION

As we saw in Chapter 8, one of the remarkable features of the human voice is that it conveys much more information than is necessary to distinguish the words spoken. We can ordinarily tell from a person's voice whether he is happy, sad or angry, if he is asking a question or making a statement of fact. We can usually tell if the speaker is a man or a woman. To a great extent, we can recognize a familiar voice and associate it with the person it belongs to.

What are the features of a speech wave that are peculiar to a particular speaker? We have only partial answers to this question. Voice "quality" is certainly important. This is affected by physiological factors, such as the size of our vocal cavities and the way our vocal cords vibrate. Other significant factors, such as speech timing and regional accent, are affected by where we were brought up, how we were educated and how our personalities find expression in our speech.

Although we know many of the features involved in distinguishing one voice from another, no automatic device has been built that comes close to rivalling the ability of human beings to recognize and identify voices. We can easily imagine applications for such a device. Law enforcement agencies, for example, are very interested in a technique for identifying persons from samples of their speech, just as they are now able to identify people by their fingerprints. Or, one might open his door or start his car by voice operated equipment, rather than relying on keys that get lost, forgotten or locked in the trunk.

SPEECH RECOGNITION

The problem of recognizing speech by machine is formidable. One might say it was impossibly difficult, were it not for the fact that we have an "existence proof" of a "machine" that is able to transform acoustic waves into sequences of phonemes and words. This highly successful speech recognizer is, of course, man himself.

Primitive automatic recognizers have been built that can identify a small vocabulary of words—the 10 digits, zero through nine, for example. These devices are fairly successful when the words are pronounced carefully, by a single speaker, with pauses between them. The problem of designing an automatic system to recognize "conversational speech"—that is, natural, continuous speech using a sizable vocabulary—is much more difficult. Its solution—if it ever is solved—will depend on a deeper understanding of the details and interdependencies of several levels of speech (as discussed in Chapter 8). Grammar, context, semantics and acoustics will all have to be considered in relation to the recognition problem.

If automatic speech recognizers ever become available

at reasonable cost, they will have many useful applications. Telephones could be automatically "dialed" simply by speaking the desired number. Even better, it might be possible to place a call just by stating the name of the party to be called, plus some identifying information to avoid reaching a different person with the same name. Another possibility is a voice operated typewriter, capable of typing letters in final form faster than a good stenographer can take dictation.

SPEECH SYNTHESIS

A "speech synthesizer" is a device that can produce intelligible speech (hopefully, of good quality) from a symbolic input, such as a sequence of phonemes. In Chapter 8, we mentioned the "Pattern-Playback" machine. This synthesizer produces speech from an input of spectral data painted on a plastic belt. A more recent synthesizer, utilizing the capabilities of a high speed digital computer, is able to produce speech from data supplied on punched cards. The input information includes such items as the desired phoneme sequence, pitch and timing.

We have already discussed the value of speech synthesis as a research tool. Through experiments with synthesized speech, we have learned a great deal about the speech wave features that are important for intelligibility. Much more remains to be learned through such experiments. In addition, if we ever perfect synthesizers that can be made to talk economically and conveniently, we will surely find important applications for them.

Earlier, we mentioned a "voice operated" typewriter. But how about a "typewriter operated voice"? A device of this sort would be of great value to people who cannot speak.

Voice outputs may very well be a useful feature of future digital computers. Combined with an input device that could recognize speech and accept spoken commands from a human operator, spoken outputs would permit direct verbal communication between man and machine.

Since we are having such pleasant dreams, we might just as well consider another remote possibility. Suppose we had an automatic language translating system, as well as a good speech synthesizer and a good speech recognizer. It would be possible, then, for two people who speak different languages to hold direct conversations—even over long distance telephone circuits—with each person speaking and hearing only his own language. Automatic devices would recognize speech in one language, translate it into a second language and prepare an input for a speech synthesizer that would "talk" in the second language.

BANDWIDTH COMPRESSION SYSTEMS

Next, let us consider the application of speech bandwidth compression systems. The *bandwidth* of a particular signal—a speech waveform, for example—is the important range of frequencies in the signal. The range of frequencies important for high quality speech is about 100 to 10,000 cps or, roughly, a bandwidth of 10,000 cps. Telephone quality speech contains only those frequencies between about 200 and 3400 cps, a bandwidth of 3200 cps. Telephone speech is quite acceptable so far as intelligibility is concerned, but voice quality is noticeably altered.

A given electrical circuit can transmit only a certain limited range of frequencies; this frequency range is called the bandwidth of the circuit. If we try sending a signal that has frequency components outside the transmission band, some frequencies will be attenuated (weakened) and lost along the way. Consequently, the received signal will not be a good replica of the transmitted signal, and the resulting distortion, if severe enough, may be unacceptable.

Suppose we have a transmission link—an undersea cable, for the sake of argument—that can carry signals within a specified bandwidth. By using appropriate electronic techniques, we can transmit many "narrow band" signals over the cable, instead of only a single "broad band" signal. Specifically, suppose our cable has a bandwidth of 4,000,000 cps (four megacycles), which happens to be about the bandwidth required for transmitting one television program. We could, at a given time, use the cable to transmit a single TV program; or we could transmit 400 high quality speech signals (each having a 10,000 cps bandwidth); or we could transmit 1250 speech signals of telephone quality. Loosely speaking, our cable system's only limitation is that the total bandwidth of all signals transmitted simultaneously cannot exceed 4,000,-000 cps.

If a way could be found to transmit speech using smaller bandwidths—say, 250 instead of 3200 cps—it would be possible to transmit many more conversations over the same cable (about 13 times more in our example). The technique of "compressing" speech into smaller than normal bandwidths is called *speech bandwidth compression.*

Such techniques offer the possibility of increasing the communication capacity of existing transmission systems, without requiring the construction of additional expensive transmission links, such as undersea cables.

Speech bandwidth compression systems have been built

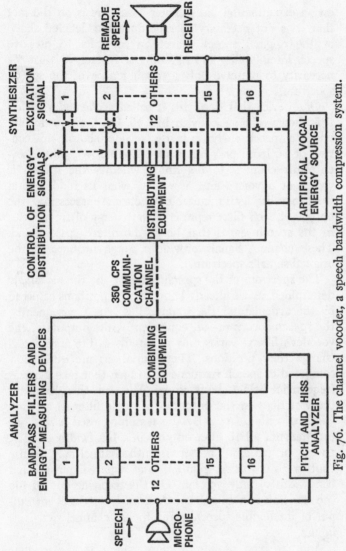

Fig. 76. The channel vocoder, a speech bandwidth compression system.

on an experimental basis. Their success rests on the fact that it is not necessary to reproduce the detailed shape of the original speech waveform in order to preserve speech intelligibility and naturalness. In fact, it is usually necessary to preserve only a rough replica of the speech spectrum.

One device that does this is called a *channel vocoder*; it is shown schematically in Fig. 76. On the transmitting end is a speech *analyzer*; in the vocoder shown, this consists of 16 band pass filters (see Chapter 8), plus a seventeenth channel to determine whether the speech is voiced or unvoiced and, if voiced, what its fundamental frequency is. With suitable electronic processing, the output of each filter represents the energy of frequencies in the speech signal that lie in the filter's "pass" band. These channel signals provide a rough measure of the original signal's spectrum.

The spectrum of the speech signal at any time is largely determined, as we already know, by the positions assumed by the articulators: the tongue, lips, etc. Consequently, the speech spectrum—or, equivalently, the outputs of the vocoder's filters—varies only as rapidly as the articulators change their positions. These variations are quite slow compared to speech frequencies; in fact, they take place at frequencies below about 20 cps. We can, then, transmit the variations in the output of a single filter in a bandwidth of only 20 cps. By the reasoning used earlier, we can transmit all 16 filter outputs in a bandwidth of 16 × 20 cps, or 320 cps. The seventeenth channel may require another 30 cps or so, giving a total required transmission bandwidth of only 350 cps. On the receiving end of the vocoder link is a speech *synthesizer*; it produces an output of intelligible speech, using the 17 channel signals as inputs.

Another type of compression system is a *resonance*

vocoder. Instead of transmitting spectral information in the form of filter channel signals, it transmits information directly about the formant frequencies (resonances) present in the speech signal. The resonance vocoder also offers considerable savings in bandwidth. Unfortunately, the quality of systems offering large bandwidth reductions is not yet good enough for use in commercial telephone communications.

In any compression system, the price paid for the more efficient use of transmission links is the greater complexity of the analyzing and synthesizing equipment such efficiency requires. Whether this complication is economically justified depends on the cost of increasing the communication capacity by other means—by laying more undersea cables, for example. Further research into the fundamental aspects of speech production and perception may lead to simple and effective methods offering even more bandwidth reduction than the vocoder systems.

ADVANCES IN NEUROPHYSIOLOGY

A greater understanding of the nervous system is the key to many puzzles about how the complex human body operates. Undoubtedly, research in neurophysiology will provide answers to some of these questions. Neurophysiology is a relatively new field and promises to be exciting and fruitful. The building block of the nervous system, the neuron, has been identified and its properties studied. We know quite a bit—though by no means all—about how nervous conduction takes place along axons. Theories have been proposed to explain synaptic transmission, but they are not completely in the realm of established fact. Beyond this—concerning how the nervous system is organized, how man learns, how he stores information in his memory, how the complex activities of the human body are controlled and coordinated—lies a fertile, relatively unexplored field for scientific research. Very possibly, further research into the nature of speech production and perception will help clarify some of these problems (and vice versa).

Increased understanding of the nervous system may have many medical and engineering applications; for example, sensory aids that couple directly to the nervous system. If a person is blind because of an eye defect, it may in the future be possible to restore vision of some sort by "connecting" an artificial eye directly to the optic nerve. Or, for people suffering damage to the cochlea, but whose auditory nerve is still intact, it may someday be possible to "connect" an artificial ear directly to the nervous system. Before sensory aids of this type can be perfected, we will have to know more about many facets of the nervous system, including how the sensory organs code information for transmission to higher levels in the nervous system.

Understanding the organization and activity at higher levels in the nervous system may lead to better techniques for relieving severe nervous disorders and for rehabilitating individuals who are now in mental institutions.

THE PATH OF SCIENTIFIC RESEARCH

While it is amusing and interesting to dream about the future, it is a very inefficient way to bring about that future. As Tennyson put it, "Science moves, but slowly, slowly, creeping on from point to point." It is the results of fundamental research that carry science forward.

There is perhaps no better way to end this book than

by quoting Georg von Békésy, 1961 Nobel Laureate in Medicine and Physiology, who has probably contributed more than any other individual to our knowledge and understanding of the hearing process. He has characterized the path of scientific research as follows:

"Of great importance in any field of research is the selection of problems to be investigated and a determination of the particular variables to be given attention. No doubt the verdict of history will be that the able scientists were those who picked out the significant problems and pursued them in the proper ways, and yet these scientists themselves would probably agree that in this phase of their work fortune played a highly important role. When a field is in its early stage of development, the selection of good problems is a more hazardous matter than later on, when some general principles have begun to be developed. Still later, when the broad framework of the science has been well established, a problem will often consist of a series of minor matters."*

He goes on to enumerate some of the forms scientific problems may take. These range from the "classical problem," which has been under attack, unsuccessfully, for a long time, to the "pseudo problem," which results from alternative definitions or methods of approach, and is not really a problem at all. Békésy warns us to beware of both the "premature problem," which is poorly formulated or not susceptible to attack, and the "unimportant problem," which is easy to formulate and easy to solve, but does not increase our fund of knowledge.

Two types of problems produce most of the worthwhile scientific results. First, the "strategic problem," which seeks data to support an intelligent choice between

---

* *Experiments in Hearing,* Georg von Békésy, McGraw-Hill Book Co., Inc., 1960, New York.

two or more basic principles or assumptions. Second, the "stimulating problem," which may open up new areas for exploration or lead to a re-examination of accepted principles. Of course, the strategic problems, when attacked and solved, lead to great steps forward. But one must not spend so much time and effort searching for strategic problems—they are very hard to come by—that he does nothing at all except search. It is really the "stimulating problem" that comprises most good research. A series of stimulating problems may, in the end, lead to a "strategic" result.

Let us hope the next few years will provide answers to many of the stimulating and strategic problems still unsolved. These answers will increase our understanding of the complex links that make up the "speech chain."

Reading List

The present book is really just an introduction to spoken communication. Listed below are a few publications that provide more information. Some are included because they present their subject matter in an easily readable form; others, marked with an asterisk, are more difficult works that treat the material in greater depth. They are suitable only for readers who have some previous knowledge of the subject.

Current research in speech and hearing is described in journals like the *Journal of the Acoustical Society of America*, the *Journal of Speech and Hearing Research, Language and Speech,* and *Acustica*.

Jones, D., *An Outline of English Phonetics* (W. Heffer & Sons, Cambridge, England, 1956).

> This is a revised edition of a book first published in 1918. Although it contains some views that are now out-dated, it is still a useful guide to articulatory phonetics.

Kaplan, H. M., *Anatomy and Physiology of Speech* (McGraw-Hill, New York, 1960).

> A useful reference work for the detailed anatomy and functioning of the vocal organs.

Miller, G. A., *Language and Communication* (McGraw-Hill, New York, 1951).

> An authoritative work on the psychology of language. Suitable for college level readers. Available in McGraw-Hill paperback.

Pierce, J. R., and David, E. E., *Man's World of Sound* (Doubleday, New York, 1958).

> A readable account of speech and hearing at about the same

level as our present volume. It covers a lot of ground and the pace is brisk. Recommended reading.*

Stevens, S. S. (editor), *Handbook of Experimental Psychology* (Wiley, New York, 1951).

An authoritative collection of review articles on the whole field of experimental psychology; articles on language, speech, hearing and neurophysiology by leading authorities in these fields. Chapters 2, 21, 25, 26, 27 and 28 are most relevant. This is the best single reference for additional information on material presented in *The Speech Chain*.

Stevens, S. S., and Davis, H., *Hearing* (Wiley, New York, 1938).*

This is an authoritative work on the psychology and physiology of hearing. It gives a comprehensive treatment of the field as it stood at the book's publication date.

* Fant, G. M. C., *Acoustic Theory of Speech Production* (Mouton, The Hague, 1960; Humanities Press, Inc., New York, 1970).

A detailed mathematical account of the acoustic theory of speech production. It has information on vocal tract configurations for various speech sounds, formant frequency patterns and speech wave and resonator analysis. Although the book presents a great deal of material, it is not easily read, even by those knowledgeable in the field.

* Fletcher, H., *Speech and Hearing in Communication* (Van Nostrand, New York, 1953).*

This is a revised edition of a book first published in 1929. It is still the best reference to much valuable data on the acoustic characteristics of speech. It requires some mathematical sophistication.

* Morse, Philip M., *Vibration and Sound*, 2nd edition (McGraw-Hill, New York, 1948).

A mathematical treatment of physical acoustics. It requires mathematical sophistication of the college level.

Liberman, A. M. et al., "Why Are Speech Spectrograms Hard to Read?" *American Annals of the Deaf*, Vol. 113, pp. 127–33, 1968.

Liberman, A. M. et al., "Perception of the Speech Code," *Psychological Review*, Vol. 74, pp. 431–61, 1967.

The above two publications provide an excellent, concise discussion of the speech process and of the way in which phonemes

---

* Out of print, but still available in many libraries.

are transformed into acoustic patterns. The second of these publications offers a more extensive treatment of the subject and gives references to the relevant literature.

Lindgren, Nilo, "Machine Recognition of Human Language," *IEEE Spectrum*, Part I, March 1965, pp. 114–36; Part II, April 1965, pp. 45–59.

An easily comprehensible discussion of the intriguing machine recognition problem is presented together with a valuable reference list.

Flanagan, J. L., "The Synthesis of Speech," *Scientific American*, Vol. 226, No. 2, pp. 48–58, February 1972.

An interesting and readable review of the current state of speech synthesis research and of the speech synthesis work of past centuries.

Index

absolute threshold, hearing 101

acoustic characteristics, speech 149

acoustic energy, speech 149

acoustic function, middle ear 89

acoustical law, Ohm's 141

acoustical resonance 46, 75, 86

action potential 127

acuity, hearing 100

Adam's apple 56

air flow, in speech production 52, 54

alveolar, place-of-articulation 73

alveolus 67

amplification, sound pressure in ear 86, 89

amplitude 22

aperiodic wave 34

arbor, terminal 124

articulation 53, 68

—, English speech sounds 69

—, manner-of- 73

—, place-of- 73, 179

—, position of tongue in 69, 71, 72, 73

—, vowels 68

articulation tests 164

artificial speech 164, 165, 195

arytenoids 57

auditory nerve 99, 138

automatic speech recognizers 195

axon 124

axon discharge 127

bandwidth 197

bandwidth compression, speech 197, 198

basilar membrane 94, 143

—, response to frequencies 94, 143

Békésy, Georg von 203

binaural hearing 117

brain   122, 133, 134
—, connection to ear   137,
                        140
breathing   54

canal, ear   86
cell, nerve   122
cell body, neuron   123
central nervous system 131
central vowel   71
cerebellum   133
cerebral cortex   133
—, and speech   137
cerebral hemispheres   133
channel vocoder   200
close front vowel   71
close back vowel   71
close vowel   71
cochlea   92
cochlear duct   94
cochlear nucleus   139
cochlear partition   92, 95
code, Morse   7
—, —, speech as a   7
communication, by speech
                        1
complex sounds, resolution
     by ear   113, 141
components, of non-
     sinusoidal waves   33
compression, of air during
     wave motion   27
—, bandwidth, speech   197
consonants, classification of
                        73
—, place-of-articulation 73
—, manner-of-articulation
     73, 178

—, recognition   171, 177,
                         190
context, and speech recogni-
     tion   8, 188, 189, 190
cords, vocal   52, 58, 59, 60,
                          76
—, —, false   58
—, —, observation of   61
cortex, cerebral   133
—, —, and speech   137
Corti, Organ of   98, 125,
                    139, 143
Corti's Arch   98
cycle of oscillation   22
cues, multiple   168

dB, see decibel
DL, see difference limen
damping   23
deaf, teaching speech to the
                        162
deafness   6
decibel   43
decibel equivalents, sound
     intensity ratios   44
—, sound pressure ratios 45
delayed feedback, effect on
     speech   6
dendrite   125
difference limen   114
diphthong   73
Direct Translator   156, 162
discharge, nerve axon   127
discrimination, frequency
                95, 114, 141
distortion, and speech recog-
     nition   186

duration, effect of, in speech
recognition 179

EEG, see electroencephalogram
ear, connection to brain
138, 139
—, frequency discrimination
by 95, 114, 141
—, inner 93
—, middle 87
—, —, acoustic function of
89
—, —, sound pressure amplification in 86, 91
—, protection from loud
sounds 91
—, resolution of complex
sounds by 141
ear canal 86
eardrum 86
effector cells 125
elasticity 21
electrical potential, in nervous system 125
electroencephalogram 136
endolymph 94
English, most frequent words
in 17
epiglottis 57
equivalents, decibel 46
erg 43
esophagus 55
eustachian tube 89
expectation, effect of, in
speech recognition 9,
188, 189, 190

false vocal cords 58
feedback, when speaking 6
—, and deafness 6
—, —, effect on speech 6
feedback loop, in hearing
organs 139
fiber, nerve 124, 129
filtered speech, experiments
183
forced vibration 24
form, linguistic 4, 14
formant 76, 83, 153, 158,
167, 171, 178
formant transition 174,
178
Fourier, Joseph 35
Fourier analysis 35
free vibration 24
frequency 22
—, formant 76, 83, 153,
158, 167, 174, 178
—, fundamental 38, 76
—, natural, see frequency,
resonant
—, and pitch 110, 113
—, resonant 25, 76, 77, 82
—, vibration 22
—, vocal cord 59, 60, 79,
80
frequency discrimination, by
the ear 95, 116, 141
frequency response 26
fricative consonants 53, 73,
158, 159, 177, 178
fundamental frequency 38,
76

glottis 57

grammar   17
"gray matter"   133

hair cells, Organs of Corti
        98, 125, 139, 143
harmonic   38, 80
Harvard Psychoacoustics Lab-
    oratory   165
Haskins Laboratories   169
hearing   86
—, binaural   117
—, and nervous system   137
—, psychology   99
—, theories of   141
hearing acuity   100
hearing organs   73
—, feedback loop in   139
hearing threshold, absolute
                                      101
—, differential   114
—, masked   116
helicotrema   92
Helmholtz, Hermann von
                                      141
hemispheres, cerebral   133
"high fidelity" systems, and
    loudness   107

identification, of speaker
                                      194
incus   88
inertia   21
inner ear   92
intelligibility of speech
                164, 182, 183
intensity, sound   42, 104
intensity, speech   149

—, and speech recognition
                                      181
intensity ratio   46
intonation   17

JND, see just noticeable dif-
    ference
just noticeable difference
                                      114

labials   73, 74
larynx   55
level, loudness   105, 108
lever principle, in auditory
    ossicles   89
limen, difference   114
linguistic organization   13
lip reading   65
liquids   73, 74
loud sounds, protection of
    middle ear from   91
loudness   105
—, and "high fidelity" sys-
    tems   107
—, neural mechanism   146
—, numerical scales   108
loudness level   106, 107
lungs   54
malleus   88
manner-of-articulation   73
masked threshold   116
masking, neural mechanism
                                      146
—, of sounds   116
mass   20
medial geniculate body   140
medulla oblongata   133
mel   111

membrane, basilar 94, 143
—, surface 126
middle ear 87
—, acoustic function 89
—, amplification in 89
modiolus 138
Morse code 7
motor nerves 131
muscles, of tongue 65
musical sounds, pitch of 113
myelin sheath 129

nasal cavity 63
nasal consonants 73, 179
nerve, auditory 99, 138
—, impulse velocity 129
nerve cells 122
—, and potassium ions 126
nerve fiber 124, 129
nerve impulse, see action potential
nerves, sensory and motor 131
nervous system, and hearing 137
—, electrical potential in 126
—, peripheral and central 130
—, signals in 126
—, and speech 134
neural mechanisms, hearing 138
—, loudness 146
—, masking 146
neuron 123
—, pulse rate 128

—, refractory period 128
—, threshold 128
neurophysiology 201
neutral vowel 71
nodes of Ranvier 129
noise, and speech recognition 182
—, white 182

Ohm's acoustical law 141
open back vowel 71
open front vowel 71
Organ of Corti 98, 125, 140, 143
organs, hearing 86
—, vocal 52, 54
oscillation 21
oscillator, spring-mass 21, 24
ossicles, auditory 87
—, —, lever principle 89
oval window, ear 87, 92

PB lists, see phonetically balanced word lists
palate 67
Pattern-Playback 169
perception, sound 99
perilymph 92
period, of vibration 22
periodic wave 34
peripheral nervous system 130
pharynx 63
phase 35
phon 107
phon scale 108

phoneme 14
—, American 15
phonetically balanced word lists 165
physics, of sound 19
physiological level, speech chain 7
pitch 110
—, complex sounds 113
—, and frequency 110
—, numerical scale 111
—, perception, telephone theory of 142
place-of-articulation 73, 179
place theory of hearing 142
plosive burst, and speech recognition 171
plosive consonants 53, 73
—, recognition 171
potassium ions, and nerve cells 126
potential, action 127
potential, electrical, in nervous system 125
power, sound 43, 103
—, speech 149
pressure, sound 41, 104
—, of speech 150
production, speech 51
propagation, of a wave 29
protection, of ear from loud sounds 91
psychoacoustics 99
puff, glottal 59, 63
pulse, nerve 128
pulse rate, neuron 129

Ranvier, nodes of 129
rarefaction, of air during wave motion 29
receptor cells 125
recognition, speech 163
—, —, and context 8, 188, 189, 191
—, —, and distortion 185
—, —, effect of filtering on 183
—, —, essential ingredients of 187
—, —, and formants 167
—, —, fricative consonants 177
—, —, and intensity 180
—, —, by machine 195
—, —, and noise 182
—, —, and plosive burst 171
—, —, and plosive consonants 171
—, —, vowels 8, 167, 179
recognizers, automatic speech 195
Reissner's membrane 94
refractory period, neuron 128
research, path of scientific 202
resonance 25
—, acoustical 46, 86
—, vocal tract 47, 62, 82
resonance theory of hearing 142
resonance vocoder 200
response, frequency 25
restoring force 21

round window, ear   94

scala tympani   92
scala vestibuli   92
scales, phon and sone   108
scientific research, path of   203
score, articulation   164
semantics   17
semi-vowels   74
sensory nerves   131
sentence   16
septum   63
sheath, myelin   129
shift, threshold   116
sidebranches, axon   124
signals, in nervous system   125
sinusoidal motion   24
society, and speech   1
sone   108
sone scale   108
sound, in air   27
—, intensity   42, 104
—, loudness   105
—, perception   99
—, physical qualities   105
—, physics of   19
—, pressure   41, 46, 104, 150
—, subjective qualities   105
—, and water waves   31
sound spectrogram   156, 158, 159, 160
sound spectrograph   156
soundwaves, in air   27
—, frequency   32
—, spectrum of   33, 76
—, velocity   32

sounds, complex, resolution by ear   113, 141
—, loud, protection of middle ear from   91
—, masking of   116
—, unvoiced, speech   73
—, voiced, speech   73
speaker identification   194
spectrogram, sound   156, 158, 159, 162
spectrograph, sound   156
spectrum, of sound waves   33, 113
—, of speech sound waves   76, 151, 152, 153, 154, 155, 156, 158, 159
—, —, long time average   152
speech, acoustic characteristics   149
—, acoustic energy   149
—, artificially produced, see synthesized speech
—, automatic, see speech, recognition by machine
—, bandwidth compression   197
—, as a code   7
—, distorted, experiments   185
—, effect of delayed feedback on   6
—, filtered, experiments   183
—, intelligibility   164, 182, 183
—, intensity level   149
—, linguistic form   13
—, and nervous system   134

—, production   51
—, —, acoustics of   75
—, recognition by machine
                             195
—, and society   1
—, spectrum of, see spectrum
    of speech sound waves
—, synthesized   164, 167,
        169, 171, 177, 178,
                179, 196
—, teaching to the deaf   162
—, and thought   134
—, visible   156
speech chain   1, 6
—, in the brain   121
speech recognition   163
—, and context 8, 188, 189,
                             190
—, and distortion   185
—, effect of filtering on   183
—, essential ingredients of
                             187
—, and formants   167
—, fricative consonants   177
—, and intensity   181
—, by machine   195
—, and noise   182
—, and plosive burst   171
—, vowels   8, 167, 179
speech recognizers, auto-
    matic   195
speech sounds, articulation of
    English   68
—, pitch of   113
—, waveshape of   79, 149
speech spectrum   76, 151,
        152, 153, 154, 155,
            156, 158, 159

speech synthesis   167, 197
speech synthesizers   167,
                    169, 196
spinal cord   131
spiral ganglion   138
spiral ligament   94
spondee words   165
spring-mass oscillator   20,
                             24
stapes   88
—, function of   89
stereophonic recording   118
stress   17
superior olivary complex
                             139
surface membrane   126
syllable   15
symbols, words as   14
synapse   124
synaptic junctions, excitatory
    and inhibitory   130
synthesizer, speech   167,
                    169, 196
systems, vibrating, properties
    of   21

telephone theory of pitch
    perception   142
tests, articulation   164
theories, hearing   141
thought, and speech   134
threshold, absolute, hearing
                             101
—, differential   114
—, masked   116
—, neuron   128
—, shift   116

tongue 51, 65
—, muscles of 66
—, position during articulation 69, 70, 71, 73
—, positions for vowels 69, 70, 71, 73
tonsils 63
trachea 55
tract, vocal 47, 48, 52, 68
transition, formant 174, 178
trapezoid body 139
tube, eustachian 89
typewriter, voice-operated, see recognizers, automatic speech

U. S. Public Health Service 101
unvoiced sounds 73

velar consonants 73
velocity, sound wave 32
vibrating systems, properties of 21
vibration 20, 21
—, free and forced 24
visible speech 156
vocal cords 52, 56, 58, 59, 60, 76
—, false 58
—, observation of 60
vocal organs 51, 54
vocal tract 48, 52, 68
—, resonances 47, 75, 81
vocoder 200, 201
voice frequency 59

voice-operated typewriter, see recognizers, automatic speech
voiced sounds 73
vowel quadrilateral 70
vowels, articulation of 68
—, cardinal 69
—, central 71
—, close 71
—, diphthong 73
—, neutral 71
—, open 71
—, pure 71
—, recognition of 167
—, spectrograms of 158
—, tongue positions for 69, 71, 72, 73

water waves, and sound 29
wavelength 32
waves, sound, frequency of 32
—, —, spectrum 33, 76
—, —, velocity of 32
waveshapes, speech sounds 80, 149
white noise 182
"white matter" 133
window, oval, ear 88, 92
—, round, ear 93
word lists, phonetically balanced 165
words, as symbols 14
—, linguistic definition 15
—, most frequent in English 17
writing, and speech 1

Speech is usually taken for granted—a tool used with great ease when one person communicates with another. Yet this common, daily activity is extremely important. The ability to communicate person to person sets humans apart from other animals, facilitates abstract reasoning and contributes significantly to the development of human societies.

Spoken communication is not a simple process. A complex chain of events links speaker to listener. The study of this speech chain involves not only physics and acoustics but also anatomy, physiology, psychology and linguistics.

THE SPEECH CHAIN is an explanation of processes involved in spoken communication, from the speaker's production of words, through transmission of sound, to the listener's perception of

(*continued on back flap*)